S $15-00

HEALTH, MIGRATION AND DEVELOPMENT

Health, Migration and Development

MICHAEL BEENSTOCK

London Business School

Gower

Published by
Gower Publishing Company Limited,
Westmead, Farnborough, Hants., England.

British Library Cataloguing in Publication Data

Beenstock, Michael
   Health, migration and development.
   1   Underdeveloped areas—Medical care
   2   Underdeveloped areas—Migration, Internal
   I   Title
   362.1'09172'4   RA393

   ISBN 0-566-00369-4

ISBN 0 566 00369 4

Printed in Great Britain by
Biddles Ltd, Guildford, Surrey

Contents

Preface   vi

1   Overview   1

PART I   STUDIES IN HEALTH

2   Nutrition and productivity   15

3   Health status and basic needs   35

4   Paying for health in a poor country   46

5   The cost of nutrition in Indonesia and the poverty line   93

PART II   STUDIES IN MIGRATION

6   Land settlement principles and the economics of transmigration   109

7   Transmigration and Indonesian economic development   143

8   The economics of shifting cultivation   154

9   Urban unemployment and the determinants of migration   162

10   Some welfare aspects of migrant-employment   170

Index   180

Preface

The research that is reported in this book is largely based on my work at the World Bank between September 1976 and September 1978. My greatest debt is therefore to the Bank which afforded me the unique opportunity of studying health and migration in some of the developing countries at first hand and to numerous members of the Bank's staff whose technical expertise was extremely constructive and supportive. Particular thanks go to Michael McGarry who led the mission to Indonesia in October-November in 1976 and to David Davies who led the mission to Mali in June-July in 1978.

Samir Basta, Alan Berg and Fred Golladay were invaluable sources of advice on the chapters concerning health and nutrition while Paul Streeten's influence provided a general background for much of this work. The research assistance in chapter 3 of Tony Phillips is gratefully acknowledged.

Finally, all errors of omission and commission are entirely my own. It should of course go without saying that none of the views expressed may be attributed to the World Bank.

Michael Beenstock
November 1979.

1 Overview

The complexity of development

Both the student and practitioner of economic development will readily agree that the transition from what westerners call economic backwardness to economic advancement is a process of perhaps unparalleled social complexity. The changes involved range across the entirety of the social, economic, administrative, cultural and political structure of the societies in transition. And within each of these dimensions it is possible to identify further matrices of interaction of which the set of economic interactions is but one. Therefore any study of the development process is bound to be incomplete and partial, an implication that is particularly applicable to an economic study such as the present.

Therefore this study somewhat arbitrarily selects two aspects of the development process for special investigation. These are the aspects of health and migration, and it should be said at the outset that the terms of reference that have been set are narrowly economic. A full study of these issues would have to be interdisciplinary which lies beyond the credentials of the present author. Instead, the objective of the exercise is to generate, clarify and extend a number of economic principles concerning health and migration in developing countries. In so doing the intention is to keep the subject matter as practical and applied as possible. However, some brief theoretical excursions are unavoidable, but even here our focus will be on essentially practical matters.

In development everything affects everything else so that to varying degrees all issues are interrelated. However, the issues of health and migration are particularly related for fairly obvious reasons. With the drift of the rural population to the urban centres the pressures on public health in the towns becomes particularly marked. Sanitary practices which were innoccuous in the rural milieu constitute a health danger in the cluttered and populous urban milieu. On the other hand it may be easier to supply public services such as water and sewerage when people are concentrated within the urban centres than when they are dispersed throughout the countryside. It may also be the case that rural-urban drift is motivated by the pull of better health prospects and public services in the cities. Clearly, relatively little is understood about these interactions.

When we speak of health in this study we shall be using the term in

1

its broadest of connotations. We shall therefore be concerned with the factors both curative and preventive that bear upon public health in developing countries. This means that we shall not only be concerned with morbidity and mortality data and the provision of hospitals, physicians etc., but also with nutritional, sanitary and educational aspects insofar as they affect health status. In this context we shall be concerned with the principles of efficient health policy where the curative and preventive linkages between various health inputs are integrated in an optimal fashion. We shall also be concerned with the benefits that improved health might generate. To some extent these considerations should serve to counterbalance the widespread view that improved health is merely a consumption benefit that the poor countries in particular cannot afford. Instead one can argue that there is an investment dimension to health which in principle at least is no different to other capital inputs. We shall also be concerned with the budgetary aspects of health planning both in the descriptive and prescriptive senses. How is health paid for, how should it be paid for?

The particular concern with the developing countries is to a large extent motivated by compassion. The bottom line of this concern is the problem of absolute poverty which threatens the quantity and quality of life in various parts of the world. Death and starvation have a compelling immediacy in a way that relatively low incomes do not. I may or may not be concerned that my fellow man is materially less well-off than myself, but I cannot be indifferent to absolute poverty. It is in this context that the study of health in developing countries becomes particularly relevant since absolute poverty is largely reflected in the absence of health in which context the limiting case is death itself. The compassionate concern for nutrition, income, employment etc. is derivative with respect to their impact upon health status. Thus, if one's primary concern is with the alleviation of absolute poverty the determination of health provides a more appropriate organising framework for analysing and combatting the problem. As we shall see below, this most probably lies at the heart of the 'basic needs' approach to economic development.

Likewise, when we speak of migration in this study we shall be deploying the term broadly. Apart from the virtually universal drift to the cities in developing countries there is also migration to and within the countryside with the settlement of new agricultural land. Indeed, this form of migration shall concern us quite considerably. We shall further be concerned with the international dimension of migration in view of the migration between developing countries and the migration from the developing countries to the developed countries. However, the two issues of health and migration will not be discussed on an integrated basis although it is implicit that the linkages between them may be quite strong.

Ideology in development

It should also be stated at the outset that this book is concerned with positive rather than normative economics. There is no prejudgement that the western industrial idiom has any intrinsic merit with respect to the various idioms in the developing countries. There can be no objective basis for comparing the welfare of modern industrial man with his nine-to-five existence, his need for cars and all the other material trappings of his civilisation, his relatively high per capita income and his enforced self-reliance following the breakdown of the extended family system with the welfare of his counterpart in the developing countries where life styles as well as per capita incomes are so different. The latter's needs are different and there is little purpose in trying to measure welfare standards by comparing per capita income levels. Indeed, such comparisons are scarcely relevant as between the developed countries. It is for this reason that health parameters are more appropriate. An annual income of $150 per capita in rural Sumatra may sound absurdly low but in practice this may not be the case in relation to local requirements. However, mean life expectancy at birth of 37 years in Mali sounds absurdly low and in practice it is a shocking figure. Health statistics are in principle a better yardstick for welfare in the context of absolute poverty alleviation than GDP statistics.

Therefore there is no ideological judgement that the developing countries should ape the western industrialised states per se. If, however, the objective is to abolish absolute poverty from the face of the world it may well be necessary in certain respects to follow in the footsteps of the western industrial societies, but it is not obviously necessary that the prevailing social orders must be overthrown to achieve this objective. With this important caveat in mind it will be important for much of what follows in this book to summarise briefly some of the prevailing and conflicting ideologies in development policy. In fact as with so many other areas of economics attitudes to development policy has had its fair share of faddishness; some would say more than its fair share. In the post war era at least four major schools of thought have evolved.

(i) *The two gap theory:*   This theory identified two major constraints on the development process in the form of capital and foreign exchange shortages. The basic view was that capital investment was necessary for sustained economic growth, however, the balance of payments constraint would prevent countries from importing the necessary capital. Thus a country might have insufficient savings, foreign exchange or both. This ideology has had a major influence on institutional assistance to developing

3

countries. For example during the 1950s the World Bank saw its role as providing the foreign exchange that was necessary for capital investment and even today it shuns both local cost finance and the finance of recurrent as opposed to capital expenditures.

The 'Two Gap' ideology largely took the supply of labour for granted in which context the ideologies were heavily influenced by the writings of W. A. Lewis[1] who argued that the rural sector would provide a virtually unlimited supply of manpower for the capital investment projects in the industrial sectors of the economy. In other words, this ideology saw the industrial route as the way forward although in principle it did not preclude capital investment in agriculture.

(ii) *The employment problem:* While the former ideology enjoyed virtually unchallenged authority in the 1950s and early 1960s, it became increasingly doubted whether the capital investment route to development was adequate. In particular towards the end of the 1960s and the early 1970s employment emerged as the principle development problem as labout market data were assembled.[2] These data indicated that there was widespread unemployment throughout the developing countries and even among the employed there was substantial 'underemployment'. Moreover, it was argued that to some extent unemployment was created by capital investment in inappropriate technologies which displaced existing employment. Thus instead of balanced growth what emerged was malignant growth which manifested itself in the form of economic dualism. In addition, it was argued that urban job creation would not necessarily alleviate urban unemployment since for every job created more than one applicant might be attracted from the rural reservoir of labour.[3] Therefore, urban unemployment alleviation could be self-defeating.

To some extent the discovery of the 'employment problem' lead to a backlash against the capital investment model. The focus instead fell increasingly on job creation even if this meant less overall economic growth. However, the initial scare that this discovery created has substantially abated in the wake of the extensive body of research undertaken into the functioning of labour markets in developing countries. It is now realised that western concepts such as unemployment do not readily translate to LDCs where people may engage in a range of informal activities[4] to make ends meet. Indeed, in the absence of unemployment benefit people cannot afford to be unemployed and instead may work extremely long hours in activities where productivity is extremely low. Moreover, the measured unemployed are frequently young people from more affluent families who are biding their time for an appropriate job that matches their educational qualifications.

(iii) *Redistribution with growth:* We have already noted that in the

1970s it was realised that there was a trade-off between employment creation and economic growth. At about the same time data were being gathered (especially by the World Bank) on the distribution of income in LDCs which indicated that the distribution of income was typically skewed in favour of the top deciles of the population. Although the evidence was extremely crude, even inconclusive, it was found that the poor might be getting worse off despite overall GNP growth in the countries concerned. This lead to the emergence of yet another ideology[5] which argued that investment projects should be concentrated among the poor so that economic growth would directly benefit the target group. Prior to this the assumption had been that the benefits of overall growth would trickle down to all strata of society in due course. Despite the absence of substantial data, the view now was that either trickle-down was not working, or if it was, it was not working fast enough.

The new school was not going to leave hostage to fortune; growth would directly be focussed upon the lowest deciles (usually the bottom 40 per cent) of the income distribution. The protagonists argued that this would jeopardise growth itself, but at a superficial level at least, it does not seem that there is any significant correlation one way or another between economic performance and the distribution of income. For example[6] the share of the lowest 40 per cent and GDP growth per capita between 1960-1977 for 14 developing countries are in fact positively correlated ($r = 0.27$) while the correlation between the former and income per capita in 1977 was barely negative ($r = -0.12$).

Unfortunately the new school confused a number of important issues and was never well conceived. First, was the distribution of income a means or an end in itself? That is was income inequality undesirable per se? A Rawlsian[7] would argue that the objective was to maximise the welfare of the worst-off social group. To this end it may be necessary to evolve an incentive structure which generates income inequalities whose justification is that it improves the lot of the poor— or what Rawls calls 'distributive justice'. In fact to reduce inequalities could well harm the prospects of the poor in a society where there are strong direct and indirect economic interdependencies between rich and poor. In this way the distribution of income is not an end but a means— an issue which the new school never clarified.

Secondly, the distinction between relative and absolute poverty became blurred. There will always be a bottom 40 per cent but the numbers of absolute poor may vary. This confusion stresses the point that the basic issue is not income distribution but absolute poverty itself.

(iv) *Basic needs:*   It is precisely in this context that the so-called 'basic needs' approach[8] to economic development can best be understood since it attempts to focus on the slippery concept of absolute

5

deprivation rather than relative deprivation. It sets as its goal the supply of a given set of basic human needs such as adequate nutrition, potable water and health care as an appropriate yardstick for economic development in the context of poverty alleviation. Conventional economic growth even amongst the poor will not necessarily lead to poverty alleviation since the individual may not be in a position to buy improved public health and other services that determine his poverty status.

Although the basic needs approach focusses on the determinants of poverty it hardly serves as a satisfactory basis for development policy. Nevertheless, it may serve as a useful starting point for the development of such a policy. In some of the chapters that follow it is argued that the common denominator of the basic human needs that have typically been identified is in fact health. Nutrition, sanitation etc. are important because of their impact upon public and private health. If they did not have this impact we should hardly be so concerned about them. Therefore, the challenge is to see how far it is possible to evolve principles of development policy where health is used as an organising framework for analysing basic needs.

This does not of course mean that all other economic issues can be ignored. On the contrary, we have already pointed out that to a Rawlesian the rest of the economy is self evidently important since the lot of the poor is not independent of others in society. It is naturally impossible to answer all questions at once and an integrated basic needs strategy would vary from country to country. At least the approach provides a perspective for considering the problem of absolute poverty, a perspective which so far has been conspicuous by its absence.

Background data

On Table 1.1 we report some background data that are germane to some of the discussions in the chapters ahead. For reasons of space the data are necessarily highly aggregative concealing fairly wide differences both within countries and between countries. The most impressive feature of the table is that the aggregate figures at least record substantial and perhaps unprecedented socio-economic progress over the period 1960-1977.[9] All the indicators point in favourable directions for the developing countries in particular although in absolute terms the figures for the low income group are depressingly low. Life expectancy is still a quarter of a century shorter than in the industrialised countries although it is increasing by about six months for every year that passes by. Also only 91 per cent of calorie requirements were consumed on average in 1974. Since this parameter must be about 110 per cent to guarantee that virtually all the population are meeting their requirements the figure

Table 1.1

Socio-economic trends

	Low income[a] Countries	Middle income[b] Countries	Industrialised[c] Countries
Life expectancy—years			
1960	42	53	69
1977	50	60	74
Population/doctor			
1960	18700	6840	820
1976	10300	4470	630
Average calorie consumption— % of requirement			
1974	91	107	130
Adult literacy rate			
1960	29	51	130
1975	36	69	99
Primary school enrolment—%			
1960	51	79	
1976	73	92	
% of population with access to safe water			
1975	28	59	
Crude birth rate per 1000			
1960	46	42	20
1977	40	35	14
Crude death rate per 1000			
1960	23	15	10
1977	15	11	9
Population growth—% p.a.			
1960-1970	2.4	2.5	1.0
1970-1977	2.3	2.6	0.8
Urban population growth—% p.a.			
1960-1970	3.4	3.7	1.8
1970-1977	4.2	4.2	1.4
Urban population—% of total			
1960	15	37	67
1975	19	47	74
Growth in GDP/capita—% p.a.			
1960-1970	1.5	3.7	4.1
1970-1977	0.9	3.5	2.3

Source: Various tables in *World Development Report, 1979*, World Bank.

Notes:
a   GDP/capita $\leqslant$ $300 in 1977
b   GDP/capita > $300
c   see ibid, page 127

implies a substantial shortfall. On the other hand (see chapter 2) the benchmarks that are used for such calculations are quite dubious.

The adult literacy figures are likely to be overstatements since they assume that people do not forget how to read once they have learned. In non-literary societies it is naturally very easy to forget one's reading skills. The very low percentage (28 per cent) of the population with access to safe water reflects the fact that only 19 per cent of the population lives in the urban areas where it is easier to supply potable water. Here too the figures should be taken with a large pinch of salt indicating no more than broad orders of magnitude.

The decline in the crude death rate has been more or less matched by declines in the crude birth rate so that the population growth rate has been roughly constant in the developing countries. However, not only has urban population growth been much higher than total population growth but also urban population growth rates have been accelerating. The process of rural-urban transition has never been more concentrated or pronounced.

A cause for concern is the deceleration in the rate of growth of income per capita during the 1970s in the low income countries mirroring the decline in the industrialised countries. How far this is due to cyclical, secular or random factors is difficult to tell at this stage. The surprising feature is that against all the odds of slow world trade growth etc. the middle income countries managed to sustain their growth rates.

Despite the intractability of the data there has been a fairly widespread manifestation of the body-count mentality where the objective is to put a figure on the numbers in absolute poverty or whose basic needs are not met. For example in its 1978 *World Development Report* the World Bank determined the numbers of absolute poor at 800 millions or 37 per cent of the total population in the developing countries. Presumably such figures apply a fairly generous benchmark for measuring absolute poverty. In this and related areas there is an obvious danger in crying wolf. Suffice it to say that a fairly widespread poverty problem exists; it is not necessary to exaggerate for the issue to be taken seriously.

The chapters ahead

The next four chapters are concerned with the areas of health, poverty and basic needs while the remaining chapters are concerned with various aspects of migration. In this sense the book naturally falls into two distinct halves.

Chapter 2 summarises what is known about the relationship between health, nutrition and productivity. This is particularly important since it is most probably inappropriate to regard expenditure on health as consumption alone. If, indeed, improved health leads to improved productivity there will be an investment aspect to take into consideration too. Unfortunately what evidence there is is rather scanty although it seems that iron deficiency anaemia is likely to be a widespread constraint on productivity. The argument that health is a pure consumption good is clearly wrong. The challenge is therefore to identify projects in which the health component has productive side effects. For example, antimalarial programmes during the harvest season which enable the farmer to harvest his crops must be regarded as a form of investment alongside irrigation, fertilisation and other conventional investment inputs.

Chapter 3 discusses how various inputs of basic needs such as nutrition, water supply and curative health care might be combined to generate the greatest health benefit for a given budgetary allocation. The purpose of this exercise is to give analytical substance to the basic needs approach to economic development using health and its determinants as an organising framework.

The chapter also sets about the econometric estimation of the determinants of health status (as measured by life expectancy) when the explanatory variables are nutrition, water supply etc. etc. The study uses a cross section of data from different countries and it is shown that the approach is a useful one.

Chapter 4 is a case study of how health and basic needs are financed in one of the poorest countries in the world, i.e. in Mali in West Africa. Despite the particular features of the Malian system it is most probably possible to make some more general inferences. For example expenditure on curative health is disproportionately large with relatively little emphasis on preventive health, the personnel budget is disproportionately large, there is over investment in the sense that recurrent costs go unfinanced so that services grind to a halt, there is excessive centralisation of administration, external aid is never free insofar as it distracts skilled personnel from their activities and creates a drain on the recurrent cost budget. These are features which are no doubt common enough in the developing countries.

On the other hand one cannot fail to be impressed by the spontaneous mobilisation of resources on a self-help basis especially in the rural areas where the people have set up maternities, clinics and drug stores. Herein lies a powerful force for improvement and a possible model for other countries. Unfortunately, this model might not work in other countries and even in Mali it is not clear how widespread these self-help schemes have proliferated.

We have already discussed the problems of measuring absolute poverty levels. In Chapter 5 an attempt is made to establish benchmark criteria by using linear programming techniques. By calculating least cost diets

9

for given nutritional objectives it is possible to arrive at an objectively based poverty line which in fact turns out to be much lower than other estimates of the poverty line when applied in the Indonesian context. The basic insight here is that the poor are forced to spend their meagre resources very carefully—or to get maximum value for money. This is the assumption behind the linear programming methodology.

The remaining chapters are concerned with migration. Chapters 6-8 are also concerned with Indonesia where the economics of the Indonesian transmigration programme are considered. This is a programme which in one form or another has been in operation for more than half a century for the organised movement (or transmigration) of people from the 'overcrowded' island of Java to the sparsely populated outer islands of the Indonesian archipelago. Transmigration settlements have usually been in jungle clearances and are based on agriculture especially of the small-holder variety.

The Indonesian transmigration programme has been and still is highly controversial. Supporters of the programme argue that population pressure in Java is so great that there really is little alternative. Opponents of the programme argue that it is costly, flies in the face of established principles of land settlement, symbolises an intellectual bankruptcy over the economic future of Indonesia and most important is prone to failure. As various press reports in the *Wall Street Journal,* the *Far Eastern Economic Review,* etc. testify, it is common knowledge that within development circles the transmigration issue has proved to be the most divisive of project areas. Perhaps one of the reasons for this is that the programme has all the glamour and sex appeal of the kind of rural development project which has gained recent popularity. The political temptation of supporting such projects is clearly great. On the other hand, at the grass roots level project staff have found it difficult to devise satisfactory projects in this area.

Chapter 6 therefore sets out some background information on Indonesia and in reviewing the literature on the subject attempts to elicit some some practical principles of land settlement. The focus of this exercise is upon the balance between spontaneous settlement and involvement by government in the settlement process. We then go on to consider how these principles might be applied in the Indonesian context. In so doing we essentially deploy a neoclassical theory of land settlement where the marginal returns to land will tend to be equated but where there might be divergences between private and social returns to settlement which would justify some kind of investment by the authorities.

This is followed in Chapter 7 by a comprehensive statement of the case against transmigration. This is of some importance since to the best of my knowledge there is no published argument of this kind despite the widespread support for such a view.

In Chapter 8 a theory is developed concerning the economics of shifting cultivation. Shifting cultivation is an interesting case where migration and land use interplay since the shifting cultivator clears land in the jungle which he then uses for perhaps three or four seasons to grow his crops until the natural fertility of the land has been depleted. He then moves on to another part of the jungle which he clears using slash and burn techniques and which he will cultivate for another four seasons. And so the process is repeated. Once cultivated plots are abandoned they are gradually reclaimed by the jungle and the natural fertilisation begins once more. After a substantial period (fifteen years or more) the jungle is ready for clearing once more and the entire cycle can be repeated.

In this way an area of land can be repeatedly used (in principle least) ad infinitum. But as we shall see the cycle is quite fragile and with population growth in particular tends to break down giving way to sedentary agriculture. Nevertheless, under a wide variety of circumstances shifting cultivation serves as an efficient form of land settlement and provides a basis of rational migration within the rainfed jungle areas. These considerations are important because the shifting cultivator has come under attack especially from official circles. Perhaps the only valid criticism is that shifting cultivation may generate adverse soil erosion or that instead of being reclaimed by the jungle the abandoned lands will degenerate into savannah which is more difficult to prepare for permanent cultivation. On the other hand, certain criticisms have been groundless while others have been overtly political. For example, the shifting cultivator is usually involved in subsistence agriculture which does not appeal to political objectives for the rural sector. He is also something of a gypsy which conflicts with administrative objectives for a stable population. In Indonesia shifting cultivation is particularly important since it is often the alternative form of land use to transmigration settlements. Since shifting cultivation requires no capital inputs beyond seed stock it is very often the most efficient form of land use in the areas concerned.

For the last two chapters of the book we move on from the Indonesian context to a more general and theoretical context. In Chapter 9 we explore the theoretical underpinnings of the highly influential theory of rural-urban migration originally suggested by Harris and Todaro (op cit.) where it is argued that migration is motivated by the difference between expected incomes in the town and rural incomes. This insight is clearly important at the empirical level. [10] The main contribution of this chapter is to rework the Harris-Todaro model on the basis of a more plausible approach to risk than was originally used. It turns out that these considerations fundamentally alter the dynamics of the migration schedule and explain why large disparities between expected urban-rural wage differentials tend to persist. The basic insight here is that agricultural workers will prefer less risky rural wage rates to their perhaps riskier urban counterparts.

In Chapter 10 we conclude with a theoretical discussion of the welfare effects of various aspects of international migration. In particular we investigate the guest-worker case which has grown to be so important in recent years. This is where workers from developing countries work for protracted but temporary periods in the developed countries and remit part of their earnings to their families back home. Indeed the importance of guest working is such that remittances are currently greater than the total aid transfer to the developing countries. The model that is developed also lends itself to the analysis of permanent emigration.

Notes

1   W. A. Lewis, 'Economic Development with Unlimited Supplies of Labour', *Manchester School*, May, 1954.
2   For example, D. Turnham and I. Jaeger, *Employment Problems in Less Developed Countries*, OECD, Paris, 1971.
3   See J. Harris and M. P. Todaro, 'Migration, Unemployment and Development; a Two Sector Analysis', *American Economic Review*, March 1970.
4   As described by D. Mazumdar, 'The Urban Informal Sector', *World Development*, 1976.
5   Expounded in H. Chenery et al., *Redistribution with Growth*, Oxford University Press, 1974.
6   Based on tables in *World Development Report*, 1979, World Bank.
7   See J. Rawls, *A Theory of Justice*, Harvard University Press, 1971.
8   See e.g., P. Streeten, 'Basic Needs: Premises and Promises', *Journal of Policy Modelling*, pp.126-146, 1979.
9   Thus endorsing the conclusion in D. Morawetz, *25 years of Economic Development*, John Hopkins University Press, 1977.
10   See e.g., R. H. Sabot, *Economic Development and Urban Migration*, Clarendon Press, Oxford, 1978.

PART I

STUDIES IN HEALTH

2 Nutrition and productivity

Introduction

The objective in this chapter is to review a series of studies that have
attempted to relate nutritional status with labour productivity.
Especially in recent years, these studies have tended to relate to developing countries where nutritional status is often poor and where it might
be argued that productivity is constrained by inadequate nutrition. If
so, an economic case could be made for improving the nutritional status
of those affected in order to raise their productivity which would depend
upon the usual criteria of acceptable rates of return etc. Investment in
improved nutrition would then be no different from investment in
general and could be appraised on the same basis.

Despite its obvious importance the social case for nutrition intervention is not reviewed here. If indeed each person is upset by the deprivation of his fellow man, then as Harberger (1978) has argued, the
improved nutritional status of the needy may be regarded as a public
good that benefits society as a whole. But these are consumption benefits and in poorer societies it would be understandable if greater weight
is attached to the productive benefits.

Although the nutrition problem in developing countries is usually
couched in terms of calorie deficiencies, e.g. Selowsky and Reutlinger
(1976), much of the recent research to correlate productivity and
nutrition has not been concerned with calories but with the effects of
iron deficiency anaemia on worker productivity. Moreover, the latter
has often been caused by various parasites which have in turn caused
bleeding and iron loss from the body. This reminds us that nutrition
cannot be considered in isolation; what is ostensibly a nutritional problem may be fundamentally related to sanitation, water supply,
education, etc. The child who is under-nourished because of loss of
nutrients due to diaorrhea and the adult who is anaemic because of
schistosomiasis are basically affected by factors that are not immediately
concerned with nutrition. However, in this review we cannot explore
these issues any further. Instead we focus on the relationship between
nutrition and productivity irrespective of the factors that determine
nutritional status, but mindful of the possibility that they may be other
than nutritional.

The main findings are:

(i) there is little evidence to suggest that productivity depends upon calorie consumption. However, there has been a dearth of research in this area, and it may well be the case that further research will produce affirmative results.

(ii) by contrast, there is some indication that iron deficiency anaemia will have an adverse effect on productivity.

(iii) the investigations have been methodologically poor. To some extent this reflects the difficulties that are inherent in the research objectives; in order to measure productivity in case studies it is often necessary to contrive what are unrealistic work contexts since more complex contexts would be methodologically intractable. The researcher in this area is faced with a Catch 22 situation, simple contexts are tractable but criticised as unrealistic while complex contexts which may be realistic produce results of debatable validity.

(iv) for the most part the statistical tests have been bivariate despite the fact that productivity depends upon a range of nutritional variables as well as other factors that are unrelated to nutrition, e.g. capital equipment. Therefore, the relationships have been incompletely specified.

(v) although the data were discrete, regression tests were not generally used. Instead the data on each variable would be split into two groups at some arbitrary level, e.g. anaemic and non-anaemic and group comparisons made. This made the tests unnecessarily sensitive to the choice of cut-off points for the group definitions, implying an implausible discontinuity in the relationship between productivity and nutrition.

(vi) despite the limited nature of the evidence the facts of life dictate that after a point poor nutritional status will constrain productivity. The research to date does not carry us much beyond this intuitive judgement.

In the second section—'Theory', we recount the theoretical linkages between nutrition and productivity focussing on the interplay between calories, protein and iron in the generation of energy by the human body. We proceed from there to discuss how in practical work situations the energy potential of the body might be related to the productivity of labour appropriately defined. In so doing, we develop the earlier approach of Becker (1965) in analysing the allocation of the individuals' time between work and leisure. Indeed, it is not self-evident that in general there should be a positive relationship between productivity and nutrition.

Finally a range of studies concerning the relationship between nutrition and productivity are reviewed. The section is divided into three parts relating to the studies on calorie deficiency, iron deficiency and deficiencies in other factors. A concluding section amplifies the findings referred to in the Introduction and identifies possible directions for future research.

Theory

Metabolism and energy generation

Metabolism can be defined as the process by which the cells convert the nutrients from food into useful energy and at the same time create new molecules for tissue synthesis and other vital compounds. The former process is called catabolism while the synthesis of new molecules is called anabolism. Since the anabolic process requires energy from the catabolic process, both proceed simultaneously.

Our present concern is mainly with energy and the catabolic process, although we note that a breakdown in the anabolic process would quite obviously threaten productivity since this failure would be associated with increased morbidity as essential cell renewal was affected. The principal nutrient for the anabolic process is protein which contains the essential amino acids while vitamins and minerals are required (as well as energy) to synthesise the protein into new tissue. Thus protein deficiency, or deficiencies in vitamins and minerals would induce failures of certain body functions which in their turn could either directly affect productivity or indirectly do so via absenteeism caused by increased morbidity.

Calories may be generated from fats, carbohydrates and protein. If the supply of calories from the first two sources is deficient, protein will tend to be broken down by the body for its calorie content at the expense of its anabolic functions. The catabolic process then dominates the anabolic process as far as protein is concerned, and anabolic failure may therefore reflect inadequate consumption of fats and carbohydrates rather than inadequate consumption of protein. It is consequently important to diagnose whether shortages of protein are directly related to protein consumption or whether they are indirectly related to inadequate calorie consumption.

The catabolic process is largely concerned with the conversion of calories into effective energy. Energy is released in the cell when the food molecules are oxidised via a complex series of bio-chemical processes. The oxygen required for the oxidation process is carried by the blood-stream from the lungs to the cells where the oxidation occurs. The oxygen-carrying capacity of blood depends on the iron containing pigment, heme, and it is for this reason that iron is so vital in the nutrition process. Other important factors in this process are riboflavin, niacin and thiamin as well as a range of vitamins and minerals. If the body is adequately supplied with these, energy generated by the catabolic process will vary directly with calorie intake and the volume of iron in the body. Therefore energy deficiency may be iron-constrained, calorie-constrained, or both. It would also be constrained by riboflavin, etc., if these were not adequately supplied.

Calories are consumed as they are used and excess calories will be stored as body fat. By contrast iron is stored within the body and may be used repeatedly; however, there is some loss of iron in defecation and through the skin cells while menstruation, pregnancy and lactation are further common sources of leakage. Iron will also be lost through haemorrhaging which in developing countries is often caused by parasitic diseases such as hookworm and schistosomiasis. Thus catabolic weakness may coincide with adequate calorie consumption if iron is deficient; the nutrition problem in developing countries cannot be simplified down to inadequate calorie consumption.

Productivity

The previous discussion suggests that an individual's energy potential (E) will be related in an imperfectly understood way to the level of iron in the body as measured, e.g. by the level of haemoglobin or haemotocrit (H), calorie (C) and protein (P) consumption per unit period, the quantity of micronutrients (M_i) in the body and a random component (u) which will vary from person to person. We may write this general relationship as :

$$E = E(H, C, P, M_i, u) \qquad (2.1)$$

The precise form of this function continues to be an area for biochemical research and it may be the case the E(　) is an adaptive process rather than some fixed law of nature. That is to say the body might have, up to a point, a way of adapting the metabolic process in order to use nutritional inputs more or less efficiently in generating energy should the need arise on a systematic basis. There are numerous cases, some less anecdotal than others, e.g. Edmunson (1976), where people seem to thrive even in the long term on diets which are significantly below the theoretical requirements that have been established, e.g. by WHO (1973). However, such an evolutionary prospect is likely to be applicable, if at all, only in the long term, and even then the scope for flexibility must be quite small. Therefore in what follows we assume that E(　) is fixed.

Although all the nutritional inputs will be important and synergistically related, figure 2.1 charts the hypothetical partial relationships between energy on the one hand and calorie consumption and iron levels on the other. For example, curve (i) plots the effects of higher calorie consumption on energy potential for given values of H, P, M_i and u. Below some point a the individual will die in which case E will be zero. As c rises above a energy potential will increase as indicated. However, after some point, c, the marginal effect of calorie consumption becomes

18

small or even zero as indicated. Thereafter, the curve reaches a plateau until 'over eating' reduces energy potential beyond point d. It is quite possible that the ac section is quite precipitate in which case a relationships between E and C will be difficult to estimate from real data.

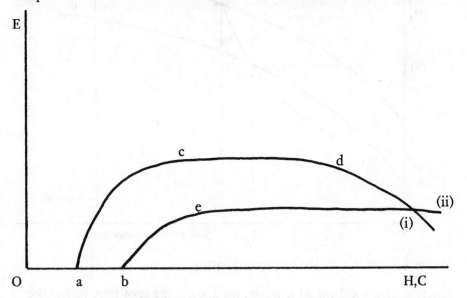

Figure 2.1, Relationship between energy and nutrition.

A similar set of considerations applies to curve (ii) which plots the relationship between energy potential and the level of iron in the body. However, in this case there is no 'over-eating' effect since the body can tolerate higher levels of iron or the surpluses are excreted from the body. Iron levels have a positive marginal effect in terms of energy potential along the be segment of curve (ii).

Given energy potential per unit period we may next hypothesise a relationship for the individual's output (Q) per unit time period. In general this will depend on the capital at the individual's disposal (K) his hours worked (T), as well as his energy potential. Thus:

$$Q = Q(K, E, T) \qquad (2.2)$$

up to a point K and E will be substitutable since it will be possible to replace capital with more effort in order to achieve a given output.

In figure 2.2, curve (i) is drawn for given values for the individual's energy potential and capital stock, and implies that as the individual spends a higher proportion of the unit period (OT) at work, marginal productivity declines, e.g. on account of fatigue. If he spends OT_1 of the unit time period at work he will produce OQ_1. Curve (ii) reflects a higher value for E and/or K. If energy potential is higher the production

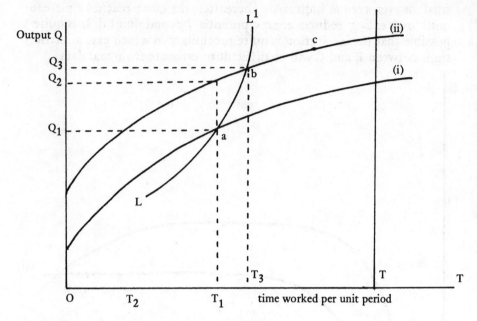

Figure 2.2 Determination of productivity

function of the individual will rise; for a lower input of time (OT_2) the individual can produce the same level of output (OQ_1). But given his production function, how much work and leisure time will the individual select? Curve LL[1] plots the individual's supply of effort and we assume that he is prepared to sacrifice leisure time in return for higher output. For example, if he can obtain OQ_1 he is prepared to devote OT_i of time to work, retaining T_1T for leisure pursuits. However, for the sake of a higher reward, OQ_3 he is prepared to sacrifice an additional T_1T_3 of leisure time. Thus in the case of curve (i) an equilibrium will be attained at a, while in the case of curve (ii) the equilibrium will be at b. If OT represents a day, i.e. the unit time period is 24 hours, in the former case daily productivity is OQ_1 while average hourly productivity is OQ_1/OT_1. In the case of curve (ii) these measures are OQ_3 and OQ_3/OT_3. Marginal productivity will be represented by the tangents at a and b.

From this analysis it follows that while a higher energy potential will raise average and marginal productivity for given time allocations between work and leisure, the equilibrium level of productivity may be reduced. On figure 2.2, the equilibrium at b implies a higher average hourly productivity than at a, although it is conceivable that the marginal productivity is lower. This solution reflects the shape of the LL[1] curve. A more elastic schedule could have intersected curve (ii) at c in which case while daily productivity is higher than at a, average hourly

20

productivity will be lower.

Thus people with low energy potentials that reflect poor levels of nutrition may choose to sacrifice leisure in order to maintain daily productivity but at a low average hourly productivity. This means that in order to disentangle the effects of nutrition on productivity from non-experimental data, it is necessary to know the nature of the trade-off between work and leisure in the allocation of the individual's time, a datum that we do not generally possess. It is also necessary to determine the individual's effective capital stock.

Taking figures 2.1 and 2.2 together implies that the production function of the individual will become insensitive to improved nutrition along the 'plateaux' on figure 2.1. Therefore, the differential between curves (i) and (ii) on figure 2.2 may reflect changes in nutritional inputs along the rising segments of curves (i) and (ii) on figure 2.1. In this context we should bear in mind that different activities will respond differently to energy potential. Brain or white collar work may require less energy than manual or blue collar work. Also, insofar as poor nutrition leads to higher morbidity, productivity would be reduced as a result of absenteeism caused by ill health. The model that has been developed in this section could be applied to this case too: the unit period would have to be conceived over a broader period, say a year. Thus days lost through sickness might be made up by working longer on other days depending upon the individual's trade-off between work and leisure.

Productivity, education and nutrition

The previous model has referred to the working adult. However, there will be an additional if indirect linkage between nutrition and productivity insofar as education eventually enhances productivity and insofar as the benefits of a child's school years are reduced by morbidity or loss of concentration that are caused by inadequate nutrition. In many developing countries school absenteeism is as high as 50 per cent as a consequence of morbidity, much of it caused by inadequate nutrition. In this paper we do not review the relationship between nutrition and schooling, nor do we review the relationship between schooling and adult productivity. In any event, relatively little work has been done on the former, although a considerable effort has gone into measuring the effects of early nutrition on later intellectual development, e.g. Srikantia (1977). But this is not quite the same thing as measuring the effects of early malnutrition on adult productivity.

Macroeconomic considerations

Our focus in this chapter is with microeconomics rather than macro economics insofar as we seek to identify, as far as it is possible, the direct relationship between nutrition and productivity. We do not consider the macroeconomic consequences of any gains in productivity that improved nutrition might bring about either in terms of higher output or in terms of longer life expectancy. Particularly, the employment implications of the productivity improvements are not discussed. There is a danger in presuming that such productivity improvements would simply be reflected in further unemployment. Alternatively, it might be more reasonable to assume that as the effective supply of labour increases the equilibrium real wage rate would tend to fall. To the extent that improved nutrition and health prolong life expectancy and consequently the working life of the individual, the same macroeconomic principles would apply.

Empirical findings

The discussion in the last section draws attention to the hypothesis that productivity is likely to depend in a fairly intricate way on calorie, protein and iron consumption. It will also depend on other nutrients but at the aggregate level and in practice these are unlikely to be major constraints on productivity. For example vitamin B_1 deficiency will induce beriberi (it will also lead to partial cessation of energy release) and the afflicted will not only lose productivity but their maintenance and upkeep costs would be a major resource burden in their own right. The same applies to blindness induced by vitamin A deficiency and goiter and cretinism induced by iodine deficiency. The productivity effects and resource costs of these nutritional factors are formidable; however, they tend to be localised rather than matters of possible global concern. Also the cures for these afflictions are well known and relatively cheap as has been discussed by Berg (1973).

There have been no comprehensive studies that attempt to relate productivity within a model that recognises the metabolic relationship between calorie, protein and iron consumption. Instead, there have been several studies whose focus has been the effect of calorie deficiency on productivity, while another set has focussed on the relationship between iron deficiency and productivity. Therefore the statistical tests that have been applied tend to run the risk of specification error which may bias the results that have been reported. This would not be a problem if iron consumption was adequate; the productivity constraint would then be calories, or conversely if calorie consumption was adequate the only productivity constraints would be iron deficiency. Insofar as both constraints are binding and iron and calorie deficiencies are correlated (as seems likely), estimates of the bivariate relationship between

22

say productivity and calorie consumption would be biased by the omission of the productivity-iron relationship.

Calories and productivity

One of the more formidable problems in experimental design in this area is the control of calories consumption and energy expenditure in the sample unless of course the sample agrees to act as guinea-pigs. This rare opportunity arose during World War II in the US when a group of conscientious objectors agreed to be guinea-pigs for a series of experiments described in Keys et al (1950). Thirty two volunteers were hired for 24 weeks and were given a diet of 1500 calories per day. As body weight fell it was found that capacity for prolonged physical work declined and that actual work performance declined as indicated on table 2.1.

Table 2.1

Weight loss and performance

Percentage change

Body weight loss	Capacity for prolonged physical work	Actual work performance
5	-	- 10
10	- 10	- 20
15	- 30	- 50
20	- 50	- 80
30	- 80	- 90
40	- 95	- 95
50	-100	-100

Unfortunately the experiment did not include a control group since to some degree work performance might have been adversely affected by the contrived work environment. Also, there was no check on the initial nutritional status of the sample; for example those who were initially over-weight might have found that their productivity improved according to the analysis contained in figure 2.1. Nor did the experiment graduate calorie consumption so that it provides evidence of a body weight relationship rather than a direct calorie-productivity relationship. Finally, the work itself can hardly be considered representative since it involved pulling on hand-pulleys until exhaustion was reached. Notwithstanding these criticisms the results show, not surprisingly, that 'starvation' diets will generate loss of weight and poorer work performance.

It is noteworthy how perceptions of calorie requirements have changed over the years and that a diet of 1500 calories per day was regarded as a starvation level when today this is about the same as what one receives under a 'health farm' regime.

While in the US during World War II, Keys et al were conducting their starvation studies, the Germans were exploring how industrial output might be increased by calorie supplementation. These results have been reported in Kraut and Muller (1946) and Table 2.2 is an example of the kind of relationship that was found.

Table 2.2

Calorie-output relationship

Calories/day	Tons of coal/Man
2800	7
3200	9.6
3800	10.0

These figures relate to averages and it is difficult to judge the overall statistical significance of the results. The data were obtained under non-experimental conditions and there was naturally no way to ascertain the energy expenditure of the sample outside the work context.

Latham and Brooks (1977) have estimated linear regression relationships between productivity in Kenya and an index of weight for height (W/H). Their hypothesis was that if W/H is low this may be taken as evidence of undernutrition. However, they do not attempt to explain the variance in the W/H ratios in their sample in terms of calorie, protein deficiency etc. Their measure of productivity was the time taken to complete a given set of tasks and the incentive was that those finishing the task early could go home from work early. Although this study is cast in a realistic work situation of road construction it seems reasonable to assume that under the incentive structure that the experiment was created, those workers who attached a high opportunity cost to their private time would attempt to finish their tasks as quickly as possible. Also throughout the experimental period simple medical treatment was provided to workers who had health difficulties. To the extent that these problems were caused by the W/H ratio, the regression results would be both inefficient and biased. The same would apply in the case of the omitted variable of the opportunity cost of time; the hope must be that it is uncorrelated with the W/H variable.

Latham and Brooks report three regression equations where the dependent variable is the time taken (in minutes) to complete a specified set of tasks and the independent variable is the ratio of weight to height (using WHO standards). The form of the regression is therefore:

$$T = a - \beta(W/H)$$

Their results are reported on Table 2.3.

Table 2.3

Task times and percentage weight for height

Case	a	β	Task
1	347	1.212	Trailer loading, ditching and sloping, wheelbarrow work, hill cut excavation.
2	367	2.018	Trailer loading
3	381	1.57	Ditching and sloping, wheelbarrow work.

Parameters on Table 2.3 have been computed from Latham & Brooks, (1977, Figs. 2-3).

All the regression equations are statistically significant, but as with the Keys et al (1950) study it is not possible to express these relationships in terms of calorie consumption levels etc. Case 2 implies that as weight for height rises by one percentage point the task of loading the trailers with earth fell by 2.018 minutes. However, all the equations are linear whereas the hypothesis contained in figure 2.1 suggests that a non-linear specification would have been more appropriate since as normal weight for height percentages are approached the productivity effect should be expected to decline at the margin. A further difficulty is that cases 1 and 3 include several different tasks; it would have been more appropriate to estimate separate regressions for each task.

Despite the highly suggestive nature of their results Latham and Brooks report that when workers were supplemented with 700 calories per day for over a 3 week period, W/H rose significantly as well as other anthropometric measures, but this had no observable effect on productivity over a 10-12 week observation period. This of course conflicts with the results reported in Table 2.3.

Tandon et al (1975) report similar correlations between a series of anthropometric measures and productivity among a sample of N. Indian road construction workers. Over a 5-hour day each worker in the sample was required to fill and then carry sand bags over a given distance. However, their bivariate linear regressions between work output and anthropometric measures were on the whole not significant with the exceptions of arm circumference for one sample and triceps fat fold for another. Since the latter sample was a combination of two sub samples in which individually the results were not significant, the reliability of the aggregated results must be in doubt and due to possible spurious correlations. In the same study productivity and calorie consumption were found to be uncorrelated.

Two other Indian studies failed to identify relationships between

25

productivity and calorie consumption. Belavady (1966) did not find any significant differences between the productivity of agricultural workers ingesting 2400 calories per day when compared with the productivity of those consuming 3000 calories per day. However, it is probable that these observations were taken from the plateau on figure 2.1, i.e. where the calories constraint is no longer binding. Satyanarayana et al (1972) did not find any significant increase in the productivity of a group of coal miners when they were given supplements of 500 calories per day. But it is possible that the lack of additional coal cars prevented the miners from increasing productivity. It is also possible that the calories constraint was not binding.

Iron-deficiency anaemia and productivity

Especially in recent years there has been a significant switch of research attention from the relationship between calorie consumption and productivity to the iron-productivity relationship. While a number of these studies have also explored the relationship between calorie consumption and productivity they did not attempt to perform multivariate investigations where both calorie and iron consumption were considered as independent variables. For the most part, therefore, what we have is a series of bivariate relationships that do not tell us too much about the overall model of productivity and nutrition.

For example, Latham and Brooks (1977) explore the effects of iron-deficiency anaemia as well as calorie consumption on productivity. They found that among an iron deficient group (when haemoglobin level is less than 13 grams per cent) task times were inversely and significantly negatively correlated with percentage weight for height (r = -0.16). However, haemoglobin and percentage weight for height were significantly positively correlated. Under such circumstances it is difficult to interpret simple correlation coefficients for productivity—what is required is the correlation coefficient between productivity and haemoglobin for given percentage weight for height. Nevertheless, Latham and Brooks found that iron supplementation brought about a marginally significant reduction in task times.

Karyadi and Basta (1973) attempted to relate endurance as indexed by the Harvard Step Text* with anaemia for a sample of Indonesian construction workers. While this test hardly represents a realistic work situation a significant relationship was found between poor endurance and moderate to severe anaemia. Incidentally the sample did not indicate any significant correlation between endurance and calorie or protein consumption, while iron deficiency anaemia was highly correlated with hook-worm infestation.

*This test involves stepping on and off a bench until exhaustion is reached.

In a follow-up study Basta and Churchill (1974) provided iron supplements for a group of plantation workers in Indonesia while a control group was provided a placebo. An income supplement was provided to the participants in the experiment to ensure their continued co-operation but since this was supplied to all of the sample the differential productivity effects between anaemic and non-anaemic workers were unlikely to be influenced although in absolute terms the supplement might have boosted productivity as a whole. Significant bivariate relationships were found between haemoglobin counts and step test scores as well as latex output of tappers in the sample prior to iron supplementation.

The post supplementation results perhaps create more problems than they solve. For example while step performance among iron-supplemented anaemic workers improved significantly by 18.5 per cent, a 15.3 per cent improvement was observed for the anaemic workers who were given a placebo. There was also a significant 4.5 per cent improvement in the performance of a non-anaemic group given iron-supplementation while no improvement was observed for a non-anaemic placebo group. From these results it is difficult to conclude anything beyond the need for further research into an independent placebo effect. Alternatively the contingency test methodology might have been inappropriate and that instead of bifurcating the sample into anaemic and non-anaemic groups, it might have been appropriate to use regression techniques with continuous observations on measures of anaemia.

Table 2.4 summarises some of Basta and Churchill's findings on the productivity effects of iron supplementation for latex tappers.

Table 2.4

Latex output/man (kg) and iron supplementation

	Before treatment	After treatment
Anaemic	20.94 (7.86)	29.78 (iron) (8.47) 25.46 (placebo) (10.88)
Non-anaemic	25.77 (9.55)	31.40 (12.57)

Standard deviations in parentheses.

The output of the anaemic and non-anaemic groups before treatment was not significantly different although the output of the non-anaemics was 23 per cent greater than the output of the anaemics. After treatment the output of all groups rose. Among the anaemics iron supplementation was associated with a 4.2 per cent improvement in output but this was not statistically significant even at $Pb = 0.2$, while there was a 21.6 per

27

cent increase in the productivity of the anaemic placebo group. Table 2.4 adds further confusion since the percentage of the iron supplemented non-anaemic group also rose (by 21.8 per cent). The results as a whole do not seem to be very conclusive. However, a significant correlation ($r = 0.56$) was found between monthly payments to latex tappers and their haemoglobin levels suggesting that the output of anaemic workers was lower since wages were based on piece-work.If these higher earnings were used to buy iron rich foods it is arguable that the causality flows from earnings to haemoglobin levels rather than the other way round.

Basta and Churchill report that prior to treatment the output of anaemic weeders was 20 per cent below that of the non-anaemics. After treatment no significant differences were found between the anaemic iron and anaemic placebo groups. Unfortunately standard deviations are not reported. The authors point out that the iron levels of the sample might have been affected by the purchase of iron rich foods with the income supplementation paid to those participating in the experiment, and that haemoglobin levels were associated with differences in output levels. Indeed, a focus on continuous observations on haemoglobin levels would have served as a more appropriate metho-dological basis for the experiment.

Although a bifurcated methodology showed significant differences in the productivity among road construction workers in the Philippines, Popkin et al (1976) regressed productivity on a range of explanatory variables which included haemoglobin levels. For example, these results implied that a one per cent increase in haemoglobin levels would raise productivity by approximately 1.5 per cent. In a follow-up study Popkin and Lim-Ybanez (1976) found significant relationships between percent-age of time worked and haemoglobin levels. A methodological advantage of these studies is that they were multivariate and allowed for the effects of age, occupational grouping, weather and remuneration on output levels. A refinement that future efforts might make is to recognize that as adequate iron levels are reached the productivity effects would tend to approach an asymptote as implied by figure 2.1.

Gardener et al (1975) found that the daily volume of tea picked by women in Sri Lanka rose with haemoglobin levels as indicated on Table 2.5. The results implying an elasticity between productivity and haemo-globin

Table 2.5

Haemoglobin level and pounds of tea picked

Haemoglobin (grams per cent)	Pounds of tea
6	21
10	31
13	37

levels of about 0.73, i.e. a one per cent increase in the latter raises the former by 0.73 per cent, or roughly half the estimate in Popkin et al (1976).

Indirect relationships between the productivity of cane cutters in Columbia and haematrocrit and haemoglobin have been reported in Spurr et al (1976). Using stepwise regression procedures they estimated the following relationship for daily productivity.

$$P = -1.962 + 0.81 \, V_{02} \, max - 0.14B + .03H$$
$$R = 0.47$$

where B denotes percentage of body fat and H represents height. V_{02} max is the maximum inspiration of air for individuals in the sample and is significantly associated with a variety of variables such as haematocrit haemoglobin and protein in a series of bivariate regression tests. Thus iron exerts an indirect influence on productivity via aerobic capacity. The study did not explore any direct effects that iron might have on the catabolic process.

Unfortunately, the standard errors of the individual regression coefficients were not reported although from the stepwise procedure that was used the coefficient on V_{02} max is likely to be highly significant. Also the determinants of V_{02} max were not investigated in a multivariate context. This study, by introducing the further dimension of aerobic capacity, underscores the need for the development of a clearly specific ergonometric model that relates physical performance to a vector of nutrients. It seems clear that simple minded bivariate correlations are inadequate for the purposes of identifying what appears to be a complex set of multivariate interactions.

Other results

In this section we review a series of studies concerning the relationship between productivity and health where there is no explicit focus on nutritional parameters per se. However, to some degree this is a disadvantage to their approach since it would have been desirable to ascertain as far as possible the interactions between nutrition, health and productivity. For example, Weisbrod and Helminiak (1977) in their examination of parasitic disease and productivity in rural St. Lucia do not specify the medical and metabolic processes by which parasitic diseases should influence energy output. The diseases that they studied were schistosomiasis, ascariasis, trichuriasis, hookworm and strongyloidiasis. Some of these parasites, schistosomiasis and hookworm, will cause internal bleeding, and as noted in some of the studies reviewed in the previous section this will be associated with iron deficiency anaemia. This suggests that it would have been appropriate to specify haemoglobin levels directly rather than to specify dummy variables for the incidence of the diseases to which these levels only in part relate. However, we note that schistosomiasis will be debilitating in other respects too, via the build-up of eggs in the body and that for practical and preliminary investigative purposes a 'reduced form' estimation procedure is preferable to 'structural' estimation.

Ascariasis in adults is unlikely to have a serious nutritional effect; instead the main problem is the damage that can be done to internal organs. By contrast, trichuriasis and strongyloidiasis cause nutritional losses. In these cases too it might have been preferable to specify nutritional status itself rather than some of its partial determinants.

Weisbrod and Helminiak regress various measures of productivity on the incidence of these parasitic diseases. Two sets of results are reported, contemporanious and lagged. The former relates current productivity to current health status, while the latter relates current productivity to lagged health status. The purpose of the lagged regressions is to determine whether the disease has a build-up effect on productivity. While this may be a plausible hypothesis for schistosomiasis its relevance for the other diseases is less clear. Also, their methodology would break down if during the lag period the individuals concerned were healed of their infection.

The results themselves do not support the build-up hypothesis. However, the tests are so crude that it would be difficult to conclude that the hypothesis was rejected either. There was some negative statistically significant relationship between daily earnings among males and the incidence of schistosomiasis, however, this particular set of results (p.154) implied that productivity was higher when the number of eggs was greater.

Unfortunately, Weisbrod and Helminiak do not report the overall statistical performance of their equations and while they find that many of the individual parameters are not significant this need not preclude the possibility that infected people may have more than one parasite, the independent variables may be colinear. However, the failure to investigate this possibility undermines some of the usefulness of their results.

In a highly aggregated context Malenbaum (1970) regressed an index of agricultural output against a variety of health status indices, literacy rates, fertilizer input and labour input in an attempt to estimate a 'health augmented' production function. The hypothesis in this context is that the productivity of a healthier labour force will be higher for given conventional factor inputs and Malenbaum takes infant mortality rates, population per physician and various other variables to augment the production function. His data are cross sections for 22 developing countries in one case, while he also explores separate cross section relationships for Mexican, Thai and Indian provinces. Unfortunately, there seems to be a misspecification in all the equations reported since the dependent variable is expressed as absolute agricultural output while the explanatory variable labour, is expressed as the percentage of the labour force engaged in agriculture instead of the absolute size of the agricultural labout force.

Malenbaum claims that his results are unlikely to be affected by simultaneous equations bias since improvements in agricultural output and economic well-being in general are unlikely to feed back onto improved health care and literacy for some time. This argument could apply to time series estimation but not, of course, to the cross section data that he happens to be examining. Moreover, his estimates are likely to be affected by the interdependence between some of the explanatory variables. For example infant mortality is likely to vary inversely with population per physician.

Notwithstanding these methodological difficulties and the highly aggregative nature of the results, the results themselves are quite suggestive and 't' values are summarised on Table **2.6**. For example

Table 2.6

't' values from Malenbaum (1970)

	22 LDCs	Mexico 1940	Mexico 1960	Thailand
Infant mortality rate	-2.7*	-2.7*	-0.3	
Population per physician	-3.8*	-1.1	-2.2*	
Dysentery, cases per 1000	-0.25			
Literacy rate		-2.0	-2.7	3.2*
% improvement in malarial death rate				0.76

*Statistically significant coefficient with correct sign

the data for the 22 developing countries support the hypothesis that as infant mortality rates (as an inverse proxy for public health status) rise, agricultural output declines. The same result was found for the 1940 Mexican data. Malenbaum failed to find supportive results using Indian data with the exception of the number of drinking wells constructed. Table 2.6 suggests that the infant mortality rate and the population per physician are important explanatory variables. However, the direction of causation cannot be satisfactorily inferred since wealthier societies will be more able to afford more doctors and interventions that reduce infant mortality.

31

Conclusion

There is little that is positive that may be concluded from the discussion in the second section—'Theory' while there is much that is of a negative nature. As an area of applied research the relationship between nutrition and productivity is inherently difficult unless simple but unrealistic experiments are organised. Common sense tells us that at some point nutrition will constrain productivity, health and even life itself, and it is difficult to see how far beyond this intuitive knowledge the studies surveyed carry us. Some of the studies report that productivity might be calorie constrained while others do not, yet all the studies on iron deficiency anaemia found that this constrained productivity when haemoglobin levels were below 13 grams per cent. Therefore, the main positive conclusion would be that iron deficiency anaemia is prima facie an important nutritional factor in the determination of productivity. If the results surveyed are representative they would imply that calories are less important than iron deficiency in programmes to stimulate productivity, a conclusion which may well conflict with conventional wisdom.

On the other hand, the studies surveyed left much to be desired on methodological grounds and for reasons given in 'Theory' the evidence cited cannot be regarded as hard either in terms of corroboration or hypothesis rejection. The main shortcoming is that the approach seems inappropriate especially in the light of the discussion in the Introduction. First productivity would be hypothesised to depend upon a range of nutritional variables—calories, iron, protein, etc.—not just a single variable since theory does not suggest this to be the case. Second, productivity depends on a range of non-nutritional factors including capital, the leisure-work trade off as described in Section I. In other words what is required is a productivity model in which nutrition plays an integral role; bivariate relationships simply fail to do justice to what is a complex situation.

Theory also tells us that as far as nutritional factors are concerned in this model, their relationship to productivity will be non-linear since it is generally agreed that it is only below some unknown point that nutritional factors begin to constrain productivity after which they do so at an increasing rate. Since nutritional data tend to be continuous, e.g. per cent weight for height, calorie consumption, haemoglobin levels, etc. etc., information is lost by grouping the data into contingency tables instead of using regression techniques where such arbitrary groupings are not necessary. The expected non-linear responses could then be estimated using multivariate regression techniques in common with statistical model building.

Bibliography

Basta, S. S., and Churchill, A., 'Iron Deficiency Anaemia and the Productivity of Adult Males in Indonesia', *World Bank Staff Working Paper No. 175,* April, 1974.

Becker, G. S., 'A Theory of the Allocation of Time', *Economic Journal,* September 1965.

Belavady, B., 'Nutrition and Efficiency in Agricultural Labourers', *Indian Journal of Medical Research,* 54, 1966.

Berg., A., *The Nutrition Factor: its Role in National Development,* The Brookings Institution, Washington DC., 1973.

Brozek, J., et al., 'Longitudinal Studies on the Effects of Malnutrition Naturitional Supplementation, and Behavioural Stimulation', *Bulletin of the Pan American Health Organisation,* 11(3), 1977.

Correa, H., *Population, Health, Nutrition and Development,* D. C. Heath and Company, Lexington, 1975.

Edmunson, W. C., *Land, Food and Work in East Java,* New England Monographs in Geography No. 4, March 1976.

Gardener, G. W., et al, 'Physical Working Capacity and Iron Deficiency Anaemia', paper presented at the 10th International Congress of Nutrition, Kyoto, Japan, August 1975.

Harberger, A., 'Basic Needs Versus Distributional Weights in Social Cost Benefit Analysis', mimeo, University of Chicago, 1978.

Irwin, M. I., et al., 'The Effects of Food Supplementation on Cognitive Development and Behaviour among Rural Guatemalan Children', Institute of Nutrition of Central America and Panama, 1977.

Keys, et al., *The Biology of Human Starvation,* University of Minnesota, Minneapolis, 1950.

Kraut, H. A., and Muller, E. A., 'Calorie Intake and Industrial Output', *Science,* 104, pp.495-497, 1946.

Latham M., and Brooks, M., 'The Relationship of Nutrition and Health to Worker Productivity in Kenya', Technical Memorandum No. 26, Transportation Department, World Bank, May 1977.

Malenbaum, W., 'Health and Productivity in Poor Areas', in *Empirical Studies in Health Economics,* H. E. Klarman (ed.), The John Hopkins Press, Baltimore and London, 1970.

Maarten, D. C., et al., 'Calorie Supplementation, Working Capacity and Productivity in Sugar Cane Workers', paper presented at the 10th International Congress of Nutrition, Kyoto, Japan, August 1975.

Popkin, B., et al., 'The Effects of Anaemia on Road Construction Worker Productivity', Department of Public Works, Philippines, February 1976.

Popkin, B., and Lim-Ybanez, M., 'Nutrition and Learning: a Study of Urban and Rural Filipino Children', Department of Public Works,

Philippines, September 1976.

Satyanarayana, K., et al., 'Nutritional Working Efficiency in Coalminers', *Indian Journal of Medical Research,* Vol. 60, December 1972.

Selowsky, M., and Reutlinger, S., *Malnutrition and Poverty: Magnitude and Policy Options,* World Bank Staff Occasional Paper No. 23, John Hopkins Press, 1976.

Spurr, G. B., et al., 'Clinical and Subclinical Malnutrition: their Influence on the Capacity to do Work', Agency for International Development, Report No. AID/CSD, May 1976.

Srikantia, S. G., 'Repercussions of Early Malnutrition in Later Intellectual Development', National Institute of Nutrition, Hyderabad, 1977.

Tandon, B. N., et al., 'Effects of Health and Nutrition Status of Road Construction Workers in Northern India on Productivity', Technical Memorandum, No. 4, Transport Research Division, World Bank, January 1975.

Weisbrod, B. A., and Helminiak, T. W., 'Parasitic Diseases and Agricultural Labour Productivity', *Economic Development and Cultural Change,* 25, April 1977.

World Health Organisation, *Energy and Protein Requirements,* Rome, 1973.

3 Health status and basic needs

Apart from drawing general attention to the importance of nutrition, water and sanitation, literacy, health care, etc., in socioeconomic development, the proponents of the so-called basic needs approach (BNA) have yet to establish workable analytical and empirical notions that development planners might be able to use. Moreover, there is still widespread disagreement as to what BNA might mean even at the broadest levels of abstraction. However, this same vagueness has afflicted other 'schools of thought' of economic development and is certainly not peculiar to BNA. For example, the previous 'discovery' that employment was a crucial ingredient to economic development hardly amounted to a workable planning strategy, while a similar fate befell the focus on income distribution and its relationship with economic growth. As time passed by, the emperor was seen to be naked after all, yet this does not seem to have dampened the spirits of the new pretenders.

The objective in this paper is therefore to set out one possible conceptualisation of BNA that planners might find a useful part of their tool-kit. Notice that our concern here is the unambitious one of dealing with a single component of the tool-kit rather than reworking it from scratch. In particular, attention is drawn to the relationships between an identified set of 'basic needs' and health status which have important planning implications in the domain of public health. These conceptual issues are described in Section A, while in Section B some econometric results are reported based on an international cross-section study which shed light on the empirical relationship between health status and basic needs.

Conceptual issues

Health as the primary human need

Development economics entails a special element of compassion. Indeed, as Harberger and others have observed there is a fundamental asymmetry in mankind's economic values; deprivation of one's fellow man is regarded with greater consternation than his opulence. We go out of our way to help a man when he is down, and it is most probably the case that international concern for the plight of the developing countries reflects this sentiment. The objective is not so much to bring the developing countries up to western living standards (nor is this desirable) but to ameliorate blatant deprivations where they exist.

Of course, everything affects everything else and the relationship between deprivation and economic activity is complex. But empathy among human beings is most probably at its greatest in the case of the deprivations associated with death, disease and ill health generally. Indeed, it is perhaps no coincidence that by and large the basic needs that have been identified reflect this compassion insofar as they have an important bearing on health status. We should not, for example, be so concerned with the provision of potable water, adequate nutrition, excreta disposal and of course medical care itself, were it not for their importance for health. As it were, health is the primary basic human need; water, nutrition, etc., are of a derivative importance.

It is not argued here that health should be the only objective of development; society itself must decide its priorities. In any case, other objectives such as economic growth will most probably improve health status both directly and indirectly, while it seems quite likely that in turn a healthier population will also be more productive. Thus objectives such as growth and health must be considered on an interdependent basis. In the meanwhile, we note that the identification of health status as the common denominator to the various basic needs that tend to be cited serves as a possible criterion for limiting the length of the list of basic needs.

The organogram illustrates the relationships implied by these observations. Notice that education (broadly conceived) may influence health status in at least two possible ways. First, teaching better standards of hygiene will tend to improve health status for given levels of basic needs. Secondly, education that raises productivity will lead to a higher attainment of basic needs which in turn will contribute to improved health status. The dotted line indicates the possibility that healthier people will have a greater capacity for learning.

Organogram of health and basic needs

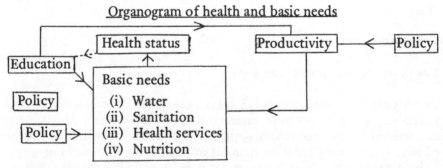

The model implicit in the organogram contains several closed loops and the areas for policy intervention are identified. This implies that policy interventions will tend to have multiplier effects and that it is possible to speak of a 'basic needs multiplier'.

For example, an intervention to improve the delivery of basic needs would raise health status. This in turn would raise productivity which in turn would have a beneficial feedback onto the delivery of basic needs. And so another round would be triggered. At the same time, there would be multiplier effects via the education loop which not only would affect productivity but also would favourable affect basic needs attainment.

The Iso-health schedule

To keep the presentation two-dimensional we assume that there are only two basic needs, say water (W) and nutrition (N). To some extent these are substitutes for each other as far as health status is concerned. It is possible to compensate for the nutritional loss due to unhealthy water supplies by additional nutritional consumption. At this stage our concern is with the underlying conceptual principles rather than the epidemiological detail, and the H schedules on fig. 3.1 map the iso-health loci associated with various combinations of basic need inputs. Thus along H_1 health status is better than it is along H_0. The schedules need not necessarily be convex to the origin, nor need they be continuous and monotonic. The configurations on fig. 3.1 are no more than illustrations. Also

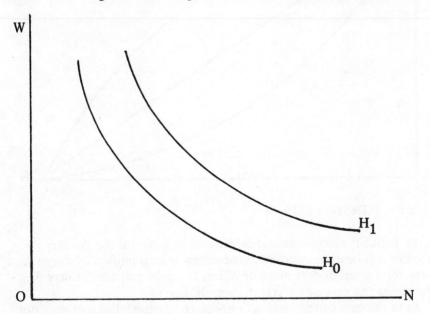

Figure 3.1 Iso-health schedules

37

because of the complexity of externalities that are inherent in the economics of public health the 'production function' that is implicit on fig. 3.1 may not be linear homogeneous. Indeed, up to a point, there could be significant increasing returns to scale since lower morbidity will itself tend to reduce the spread of contageous diseases.

Delivery linkages

The shape of the iso-health schedules will reflect the nature of the impact linkages regarding basic needs. However, there may also be delivery linkages in so far as economies can be achieved by combining different services. Once again our focus here is on principles and no attempt is made to enter into technical detail. These possibilities are characterised on fig. 3.2. A given budget line is assumed (BB^1), either OB of W can be supplied or OB^1 of N. If there are no delivery linkages the delivery frontier at this scale will be a straight line as described by

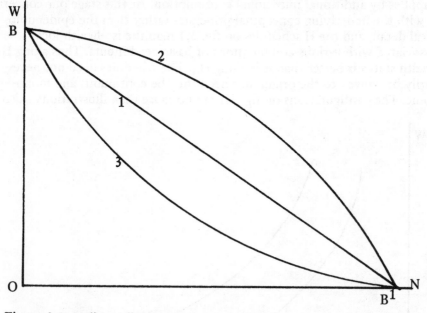

Figure 3.2 Delivery linkages

curve 1. But if economies in delivery can be achieved the delivery frontier will become concave to the origin as exemplified by curve 2, since for a given budget more of W and N can be provided. Curve 3 represents the case of adverse delivery linkages.

As in the case of the impact linkages, the delivery linkages may not be linear homogeneous. The economies or diseconomies of scale will

depend on the precise contexts for which the delivery of basic needs is
planned.

Towards a theory of basic needs

The impact and delivery linkages may be combined in a programme that
maximises the objectives of BNA. In this context this amounts to maxi-
mising health status given the constraints that have been discussed. The
problem is simple enough and its solution is characterised on fig. 3.3.
Health status is maximised at x so that given the budget constraint
OW* of water services are provided and ON* of nutrition. This constitutes an efficient allocation of basic needs with respect to the impact
and delivery linkages.

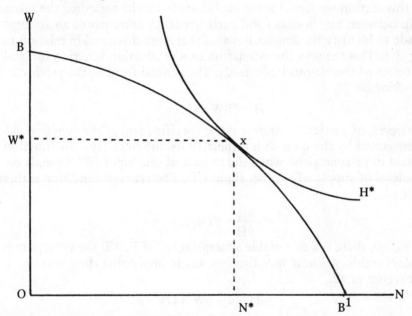

Figure 3.3 The basic needs solution

It should be recalled that this is only part of a wider optimisation
programme. In terms of the organogram we have only been exploring
the planning principles regarding the relationship between basic needs
and health status. More generally, it would be important to take into
account the relationships incorporated in the productivity loop.

Disaggregation

For expositional purposes we have postulated a single index for health

39

status. While in principle such an index could be constructed, this hardly seems desirable. In practice it will be appropriate to identify a series of indices with reference to different maladies and socioeconomic groups.

Likewise, the problem itself is clearly not two-dimensional, nor is it timeless. There are several basic needs inputs and their impacts are likely to be distributed over time. Nevertheless, the principles of optimisation will be the same; only the details will be different.

Some empirical results

The model

In this section we report some econometric results regarding the relationship between health status and basic needs. In other words an attempt is made to identify the impact linkages that were discussed in relation to fig. 3.1. This requires the estimation of a production function for health in terms of the various basic needs. The general form of the production function is:

$$H = H(W, N, ...)$$

However, of particular interest is the specific form of the function that is suggested by the data with respect to its non-linearity. The function is said to be synergistic when the impact of one input (W) depends on the level of supply of another input (N). The synergy condition is therefore :

$$\frac{\partial H}{\partial H} = F(N, ...)$$

If $F_N > 0$, there is a favourable synergism and if $F_N < 0$ the synergism is unfavourable. A linear specification would imply that there was no synergism at all.

$$H = a + bW + cN + ...$$

In this case the iso-health schedules would be linear too. One of the many synergistic specifications is

$$H = aW^b N^c ...$$

since in this case

$$\frac{\partial H}{\partial H} = abW^{b-1} N^c ...$$

i.e., the derivative with respect to W depends on N.

The data

The data were drawn from the World Bank's socioeconomic data bank unless otherwise stated. All data refer to 1970 and were drawn from an international cross-section based on the countries listed in Table 3.1.

Table 3.1
Sample of countries

Cyprus	Somalia	Bolivia	Afghanistan
Morocco	Togo	Brazil	Burma
Congo	Uganda	Chile	India
Ghana	Dom. Republic	Colombia	Nepal
Ivory Coast	El Salvador	Guyana	Pakistan
Kenya	Honduras	Paraguay	Indonesia
Liberia	Jamaica	Uruguay	S. Korea
Mauritania	Panama	Iraq	Singapore
Sierra Leone	Argentina	S. Arabia	Thailand

The country selection reflects the availability of data for the following variables.

	Variable	Source
H	Life expectancy at birth (years)	Data Bank (IBRD)
D	Population per doctor	,,
C	Per capita calorie consumption (% of WHO-FAO requirements)	,,
LIT	Adult literacy rate %	,,
HOS	Population per hospital bed	,,
PROT	Daily protein consumption (gm)	,,
HIPROT	of which animal and pulse	,,
NURSE	Population per nurse	,,
W	Population served with potable water %	WHO
X	Population served with excreta disposal %	,,
X^1	Log X, etc.	,,

Thus H is used as an index of health status while all the remaining variables are possibly explanatory variables. A correlation matrix of these variables is provided in Table 3.2 which indicates a satisfactory degree of independence between the independent variables.

Table 3.2

Correlation matrix of basic needs

	H	D	C	LIT	HOS	PROT	HIPROT	NURSE	W	X
H	1.0000	-0.6636**	0.5792**	0.9500**	-0.4295	0.6340**	0.6774**	-0.3970	0.7877**	0.7933**
D	-0.6636**	1.0000	-0.3029	-0.6443**	0.7226**	-0.4315	-0.4261	0.7542**	-0.5842**	-0.5605*
C	0.5792**	-0.3029	1.0000	0.5968**	-0.1929	0.6138**	0.5828**	-0.2391	0.2602	0.3453
LIT	0.9500**	-0.6443**	0.5968**	1.0000	-0.4222	0.5811**	0.6413**	-0.3709	0.7050**	0.6851**
HOS	-0.4295	0.7226**	-0.1929	-0.4222	1.0000	-0.1546	-0.3308	0.8032**	-0.4692*	-0.4910*
PROT	0.6340**	-0.4315	0.6138**	0.5811**	-0.1546	1.0000	0.8663**	-0.3370	0.5303*	0.4896*
HIPROT	0.6774**	-0.4261	0.5828**	0.6413**	-0.3308	0.8663**	1.0000	-0.3460	0.5372*	0.5975**
NURSE	-0.3970	0.7542**	-0.2391	-0.3709	0.8032**	-0.3370	-0.3460	1.0000	-0.4540*	-0.4156
W	0.7877**	-0.5842**	0.2602	0.7050**	-0.4692*	0.5303*	0.5372*	-0.4540*	1.0000	0.8325**
X	0.7933**	-0.5605*	0.3453	0.6851**	-0.4910*	0.4896*	0.5975**	-0.4156	0.8325**	1.0000

*-Signif. Pb .01
**-Signif. Pb .001

42

Results

Some results are reported in Table 3.3 on p.44. We begin by reporting the results of a stepwise regression with a semi logarithmic specification. The order of the explanatory variables reflects the selection of the programme itself.

$$H = -10.19 - 2.15D^1 + 5.3LIT^1 + 11.57C^1 + 2.22X^1 + .001HOS$$
$$\quad\quad\quad (3.05) \quad\quad (3.57) \quad\quad (1.42) \quad\quad (2.48) \quad\quad (1.54)$$

$$+ .073PROT + .635W^1$$
$$\quad (1.27) \quad\quad\quad (0.64)$$

Standard error (σ) = 3.837

$\overline{R}^2 = 0.89$

't' values in parentheses

The programme failed to include $NURSE^1$ and $HIPROT^1$ since they had zero F values. With the exception of HOS^1, all variables have the appropriate sign and the coefficients of D^1, LIT^1 and X^1 are significant. However, although they have the expected sign, the coefficients on C^1, $PROT^1$ and W^1 are not significant at the 95 per cent level although quite clearly the equation as a whole is highly significant.

Table 3.3 reports some further results which attempt to determine the appropriate synergistic specification as reflected in the sample. This is achieved by experimenting with alternative multiplicative arrangements of the explanatory variables. Thus in the first equation the dependent variable is logarithmic while the independent variables are linear. In equation 2 the specification is reversed; the independent variables are logarithmic while the dependent variable is not. In equation 3 both sets of variables are logarithmic, while in equation 4 the entire specification is linear. Clearly, further specifications are worthy of investigation. In particular, groups of explanatory variables might belong to the same synergy while other variables might belong to a separate synergy and therefore to a separate group. For example if X_1 and X_2 belong to one synergy, X_3 and X_4 belong to another while all variables are synergistically related to X_5, the specification would be:

$$H = AX_5^a(X_1^b X_2^c + X_3^d X_4^e)$$

However, investigation of such complex possibilities will have to await a later occasion.

The results reported on Table 3.3 are intended to be indicative of what further investigation might produce. They are not to be regarded as final or optimal. Nevertheless, they are highly suggestive as they stand with the explanatory variables representing the main basic needs of nutrition, water, sanitation, health care and education. Clearly further indices might be appropriate, but the results strongly support the hypothesis that health status is determined by the supply of basic human needs.

Table 3.3

Regression results

Dependent variable	LIT	C	D	W	X	σ	$\bar{R}^2$
1 H^1	.00416 (6.7)	.00238 (1.9)	- .001 (2.68)	.00042 (0.7)	.001 (1.96)	0.0675	0.907
2 H	5.029^1 (3.3)	16.713^1 (2.2)	-3.237^1 (3.35)	0.413^1 (0.41)	1.633^1 (1.87)	3.956	0.883
3 H^1	0.1041^1 (3.88)	0.26^1 (1.98)	-0.0642^1 (3.78)	$.0085^1$ (0.49)	$.0276^1$ (1.81)	0.0697^1	0.901
4 H	0.2126 (7.6)	0.1136 (1.92)	- .00004 (1.2)	.06533 (2.14)	0.05251 (2.22)	2.67	0.943
5 H^1	0.0043 (7.4)	0.00268 (2.2)	-0.001 (3.48)		0.00115 (2.5)	0.0671	0.908

Indeed, it is because of this causality that they are to be regarded as basic. Further investigation is likely to strengthen the results obtained so far.

In terms of $\bar{R}^2$ equation 4 performs the best suggesting that the basic model is linear rather than multiplicative in terms of the explanatory variables. Only the double logarithmic specification implies a full synergy between the explanatory variables (equation 3), yet this has a significantly inferior performance. Future research might investigate two aspects in this context. First, because the dependent variable is likely to have an asymptotic and therefore non-linear relationship with the independent variables, irrespective of the synergistic pattern, it will be necessary to find the appropriate non-linear functional form. Secondly, it will be necessary to estimate the synergistic pattern itself. The present results do not attempt to cover these separate estimation problems, in which case the linear model may not be optimal in terms of the data.

The parameter estimates in equation 3 may be regarded as elasticities. Thus, e.g., if the proportion of the population with potable water rises by one per cent, life expectancy will rise by 0.0085 per cent. The largest elasticity is associated with the nutrition variable (C) while the literacy rate (LIT) has an elasticity of 0.1041. To obtain the same increase in life expectancy via an increase in the proportion of the population with excreta disposal (X) as by an increase in average per capita calorie consumption (C), the percentage increase in the former would have to be 9.42 (= 0.26/0.0276) times the increase in the latter.

Concluding remarks

It is inevitable that in an international cross section study data problems may be severe. First, although the data from the different countries are supposed to be comparable they may in practice not be strictly comparable. For statistical purposes the key question is whether any data errors are randomly distributed or not. Secondly, cultural and other factors may influence health status and these will constitute omitted variables. For our present purposes what matters is whether these variables are correlated with the explanatory variables in which case specification bias would arise. The statistical significance of the coefficients suggests that the former is unlikely, while to avoid the latter it would clearly be desirable to perform the same exercise within a given country where cultural and related factors are likely to be more homogeneous. Indeed, this could be the focus of future research.

4   Paying for health in a poor country

The institutional background

In Mali resources are mobilised for expenditures on health at several different levels and through a variety of institutions. Naturally, by far the most important of these are the expenditures that come under the State Budget and which are expended by the Ministère de la Santé Publique (MSP). For example in 1978 the State Budget provided for expenditure by MSP of MF4518 million or $1.63 per capita, which compares with per capita GNP of approximately $100. However, an unquantifiable but significant volume of resources are mobilised under a range of different budgets so that it can safely be said that considerably more than 1.63 per cent of GNP is expended on health.

Table 4.1 lists the principal budgetary institutions in Mali where health expenditures are involved.

Table 4.1

Budgetary institutions for health

1 National Budget   )
2 Regional Budget   ) State Budget
3 Pharmacie Populaire
4 Parastatal Enterprises
5 Social Security
6 Official aid
7 Unofficial aid
8 Municipality
9 Co-operatives

The State Budget

The State Budget has two components, the National Budget and the Regional Budget. In the case of MSP for former is the most important; in 1978 it accounted for 78.6 per cent of the State Budget, while for the State Budget as a whole the National Budget accounted for 89 per cent. The National Budget is responsible for expenditures of state-wide importance although in practice it sometimes appears that the division of responsibility between the National and Regional Budgets is quite arbitrary. Thus the National Budget of MSP covers the regional hospitals as well as investment in the maternity clinics at the cercle level. It also covers the Service des Grandes Endémies, the Lutte Antituberculeuse, the Pharmacie d'Approvisionment and the training of nurses and midwives. However, the École de Médecine et de Pharmacie comes under the budget of the Ministère de l'Éducation Nationale, so that medical training is not the responsibility of a single ministry.

The Regional Budget is responsible for the PMI[2], AM[3] and the Service d'Hygiene[4]. Since the Service des Grandes Endémies[5] and the Lutte Antituberculeuse are not administered along the conventional administrative structure (state-regional-cercle-arrondissement-village), it would seem that the National Budget of MSP operates down to the level of the region, while the National Budget operates down from the level of the cercle.

It is emphasised, however, that the distinction between the Regional and National Budgets is largely artificial and that the Regional Budget enjoys no fiscale independence. Indeed, this lack of autonomy reflects the political economy upon which Mali has become increasingly dependent during the post-colonial era. Whereas once revenues could be raised at the cercle level for local use, the tendency has been to centralise all revenues under the State Budget reflecting the political need to finance the consumption requirements of the salariat. Thus fiscal resource generation has increasingly been allocated to pay for the salaries of the functionnaires at the state level at the expense of investment at the local level. This centralisation has evolved on a de facto basis and has not been enforced by law. On the contrary, the fiscal autonomy of the cercle exists de jure, but this autonomy has been lost through political patronage at the local level which has been despensed from the centre.

Thus for fiscal purposes it seems more appropriate to focus on the State Budget rather than to distinguish between the Regional and National Budgets, the latter being rumps of the past. This may be illustrated in the context of the budgetary decision taking the budget of MSP as an example. The Directeur Régional de la Santé sends his budget proposal to the Sous-ordinance (regional branch) of the Ministry of Finance covering the items that are under his responsibility. This budget will include a minimal amount of revenues from payments for confinements at the maternity centres. It will not include drug expenditures since these are handled by the Pharmacie d'Approvisionment[6] which comes under the National Budget.

The Sous-ordinance will receive budget estimates from other departments which together will make up the expenditure side of the Regional Budget. The revenue side consists of receipts from the Minimum Fiscal (poll tax), cattle taxes, vehicle taxes, etc. Once again the allocation of revenues between the Regional and National Budgets seems to be quite arbitrary since it is not obvious why poll taxes appear under the former

47

while direct and indirect tax revenues appear under the latter. Indeed, 40 per cent of the Minimum Fiscal is allocated to the National Budget with the remainder being allocated to the Regional Budget. Since at the end of the budgetary accounting the two budgets are consolidated, this proportion is entirely arbitrary.

Under the direction of the regional governor the Sous-ordinances submit their proposals to the Ministry of Finance. At the same time the Direction Nationale de MSP submits its component of the National Budget to the Ministry of Finance. Notice that this means that the Direction Nationale is unaware of the requirements of the Direction Régionale. Since, by and large, the Direction Nationale plans investment at the regional as well as the national levels, while the Direction Regionale undertakes the recurrent cost implications of the former investments, there is a built-in dichotomy between the planning of recurrent expenditures and their associated investments at the level of the cercle.

Having received the budget submissions, a Committee of Arbitration is convened which includes the Ministry of Finance, the Ministry of Planning and the ministry whose budget proposal is being reviewed. In the case of health this would be MSP; but this would primarily be for the National Budget. After this stage the State Budget as a whole is submitted to the Council of the Government for political approval. Naturally during this review process the original budget submissions may be substantially modified.

Table 4.2

The Regional Budget in 1978
(millions of MF)

Region	Revenue	Expenditure	Balance
Kayes	637.1	1019.8	- 382.7
Bamako	1360.4	2055.2	- 694.8
Sikasso	1142.0	1027.5	114.5
Segou	891.3	974.9	- 83.6
Mopti	1179.4	805.5	373.9
Gao	410.0	847.3	- 437.3
Total	5620.2	6730.2	-1110.0

Source: Budget d'État 1978. Direction Nationale du Budget.

The revenues of the Regional Budgets are effectively put into one pot and are used to finance the overall State Budget. This will involve the transfer of funds between regions as well as the transfer of revenues in National Budget to the Regional Budget. Table 4.2 records the provisions for the Regional Budget in 1978 for Mali's six regions[7] and indicates that resources are being transferred from Mopti and Sikasso to the other regions, especially Bamako. In addition to these resources, the regions were to receive 1,100m MF from the National Budget. Since this regional allocation is decided in Bamako it follows that the Regional Budget has no autonomy at all and that the distinction between the Regional and National Budgets is no more than nominal.

Pharmacie Populaire and finance of the parastatals

The Pharmacie Populaire[8] provides the majority of drugs in Mali. Whereas in 1977 the drug purchases of the Pharmacie d'Approvisionne-ment amounted to MF 1,000m, the drug sales of the Pharmacie Popu-laire totalled MF 3,256.3m. Thus Malians have been spending annually about $1.23 on drugs purchased from the Pharmacie Populaire which compares with the per capita expenditure of $1.63 in the State Budget. When the drugs of the Pharmacie d'Approvisionnement are entered into the calculation, Malians have been spending an average of $1.61 per year on drugs, or 56 per cent of the total health expenditures reviewed so far.

The Pharmacie Populaire's gross profit margin is 23.7 per cent, but when costs and taxes are taken into consideration the net return has been calculated at 3.7 per cent. Thus the population pays the full cost of the drugs they purchase at the 332 vending points that the Pharmacie Populaire sponsors. Indeed, since the average rate of duty on drug imports is 13.6 per cent, while additional taxes of 1.1 per cent are imposed, the population pays considerably more than the full costs of the drugs they purchase.

In addition to its drug sales the Pharmacie Populaire runs a medical diagnostic centre (Centre de Diagnostic et de Traitement) in Bamako with an annual turnover of MF 42.7m, and two dental centres in Bamako with a combined turnover of MF 31.3m. The net profit margin on the former is about 3.3 per cent while the profit margin on dental activities is about 23.3 per cent.

The Pharmacie Populaire is a public enterprise which is therefore answerable to the Ministère de Tutelle des Sociétés et Enterprises d'État. However, public enterprises do not generally received resources from the State Budget; they either generate them internally or they borrow from the banking system. Therefore, the public enterprises are able to run deficits and the Pharmacie Populaire has recently emerged from a period of financial stress. The public enterprises and the private sector more generally have an indirect access to the French capital market since the Malian franc is de facto fully convertible with the French franc. Thus the Central Bank of Mali runs an Operations Account with the French treasury which effectively means that the French accept the balance of payments deficits of the Malians. This relationship is reflected in the figures on Table 4.3 where the balance on the Operations Account is closely correlated with the balance of payments which in turn is associated with the credit discounted by the Central Bank as might be expected from a monetary analysis of the balance of payments. Finally the rediscounting of the Central Bank reflects the credit to the public enterprises. It is through this channel (the 'French connection') that Malian public enterprises, including the Pharmacie Populaire, have access to the French capital market.

Table 4.3

Monetary analysis (millions of MF)

	1974	1975	1976	1977
Bank credit to public enterprises (stock)	49900	77300	94200	92800
Credit rediscounted by Central Bank (stock)	42100	64800	81700	74700
Other bank credit (stock)	19800	24900	28400	30300
Balance of payments	-16832	-26813	-16333	6535
Overall balance on Operations Account	-15831	-21312	-15673	8241

Source: Central Bank of Mali.

To some extent the same applies to the central government when it obtains credit from the central bank. However, the French government constrains the central bank to advance money to the government up to a ceiling equal to 15 per cent of the tax revenues of the previous year. This places an upper limit on the resource transfer via the Operations Account insofar as the central government's financial operations are concerned. Invariably the Malian government finds itself up against this ceiling but its recent concerted efforts to improve its tax collection (by 1977 tax revenues were expected to have grown by 60 per cent over a two year period) have substantially raised this ceiling. As for other forms of bank credit, the French have been attempting to establish monetary guide-lines for the Central Bank of Mali.

While the Pharmacie Populaire has experienced financial difficulty in the past, it is most probably fair to say that while it has benefitted from this 'French connection' its performance relative to the other parastatals has been good. However, it is difficult to judge how far this has been due to managerial factors on the one hand and to the government's pricing policies on the other. The Pharmacie Populaire has been relatively free from price controls so that it could charge to cover its costs; the politics of food pricing are considerably more complex than the politics of drug pricing. Indeed, in 1978 the Pharmacie Populaire further raised its prices by 15 per cent.

The co-operatives and other independent budgets

Mali has had a long tradition of co-operation at the village level which has played an important role in the political and economic development of the country. Indeed, the Keita regime[9] propagated the view that Malians had an historical inclination towards socialism which has survived the French colonisation and which could provide the political basis for its future economic and social development. It is most probably the case, however, that the policy of fostering the establishment of co-operatives usurped an underlying co-operative spirit that indeed prevailed in the country, especially at the village level. The state trading corporations, whose policy has largely been to purchase agricultural output at artificially low prices from the co-operatives, have effectively been transfering resources from the countryside to the towns at the expense of the peasantry and to the advantage of the salariat or fonctionnaire class. In fact, this has emerged as a critical feature in the nation's political economy which to some extent may have soured the indigenous co-operative spirit in the rural areas especially in relation to co-operatives that are organised from outside the village arrondissement.

Nevertheless, especially in the regions of Sikasso and Bamako south of the Niger, there is substantial evidence of village co-operation in the context of health and the social services more generally. Perhaps the most extensive area of involvement concerns the purchase of drugs at a 15 per cent rebate from the Pharmacie Populaire and there are currently (mid 1978) 279 outlets for drugs at the village and arrondissement level most of which are sponsored by co-operatives. In 1977 these outlets accounted for about MF 182 millions or 5½ per cent of the total sales of the Pharmacie Populaire. The co-operatives sell these drugs at the official price so that they make a margin of 15 per cent on their sales. (New outlets receive a 20 per cent rebate during the first year.) The profits are ploughed back into the general activities of the co-operative and the co-operatives themselves are required to invest 20 per cent of their total profits in the social services.

The following organogram summarises the administrative hierarchy of co-operation in Mali. As far as health is concerned the FGR and to some extent the CAC are the principal points of participation. Unfortunately, comprehensive data on the expenditures of the CAC and FGR are not available so it is not possible to estimate the health budget from this source. But the resource contributions are not limited to money; and there is extensive evidence of self help in the construction of wells, dispensaries, operating blocks and maternity centres. For example in the Sikasso region where a network of rural maternities is being established, virtually no resources are being consumed out of the State Budget. The building materials are bought with funds from the FGR, CAC and the Association de Parents des Élèves (APE), the labour is largely supplied voluntarily by the community, bedding is supplied and made by the local women's groups, the training of the matronnes is financed by the villagers (i.e., while she is away at the cercle the villagers look after her fields, etc.), basic equipment is provided by UNICEF, the women pay MF 300 for their confinement and bring with them food, sheets, etc., and the matronnes are paid MF 10,000 per month out of the proceeds from FGR drug sales. At no stage therefore are state funds or resources involved. Where it is practiced, e.g., Baguineda (in the Bamako region) the training of animateurs and secouristes[10] are financed on a similar basis.

Organogram of co-operative structure

Ministère du Développement Rural
|
Direction Nationale de la Coopération
|
Direction Régionale (the Regional level)
|
Centre d'Associations Coopératives (CAC) (Cercle level)
|
Fedération de Groupements Ruraux (FGR)
(Arrondissement and village levels)

For example in the cercle of Kadiolo[11] (Sikasso region) APE spent MF 7.6 millions on health in 1977 out of a total of MF 49.7 millions (on an ambulance and an operating block) while CAC contributed approximately MF 2 millions. In the arrondissement of Niéna[12] FGR spent MF 2.2 millions in 1977 on health out of a total of MF 31.3 millions, while in the cercle of Koutiala there is similar evidence of local resource mobilisation for an X-ray block, a paediatric centre, a hangar for a prefabricated dispensary and a water reservoir.

All the previous observations have related to the region of Sikasso. In the Bamako region there was similar evidence of community participation, but in the other regions there was very little evidence of such activity. In the Mopti region in the arrondissement of Sangha the community were constructing a rural maternity, while at Samé in the Kayes region the FGR were running a dispensary. For some reason, possibly economic, possibly cultural, village co-operation for health was concentrated in the south-east of the country. One explanation is that the Malinke are an especially co-operative people; another is that the Sikassoise in particular are relatively prosperous and can afford to raise the necessary funds. However, the data in Appendix 4 do not

52

support this latter hypothesis.

Another independent budget is that of the municipality which raises revenues for local use from its citizens. However, the municipality does not generally involve itself in health and related activities.

Health and basic needs in the national plan

Since independence, Mali has continued the colonial policy of indicative economic planning under the direction of the Ministère du Plan et de la Statistique. There have been three plans to date.

  (i) Five Year Plan; 1961-1965.
 (ii) Three Year Programme for Financial and Economic
        Recovery; 1970-1972.
(iii) Five Year Plan; 1974-1978.

At the present time a further five year plan is being proposed, but it is unlikely that it will run from 1979-1983 since so far it is not sufficiently advanced. The first plan was conceived in the spirit that followed the declaration of independence. It was largely prepared with French assistance and its ambitiousness seems to have set the style for the subsequent plans. The Recovery Programme was a response by the new regime to the economic and financial imbalances that had developed during the Keita regime. However, this was thwarted by the Great Drought in the early 1970s. Finally, the most recent plan responded to the post drought recovery and like its precursors laid extensive emphasis on the agricultural sector and the development of transportation infrastructure. In this section, however, we explore the role of health in these plans, especially the latest five year plan.

The earlier plans

Mali's economic plans have been loosely conceived and in many respects have been little more than shopping lists of investments for which foreign assistance would be sought. In view of the unpredictability of such assistance it has often been the case that outcomes have borne little resemblance to the plan itself. Usually the amount of external assistance was overestimated and in many cases donors preferred projects that were not included in the plan. Table 4.4 reports the importance of external financial assistance in planned investment and indicates that Mali's planners have become increasingly dependent in this regard. The more Mali becomes dependent on external finance the less predictable will its execution programme become. Thus in the most recent plan Malians intended to provide only 10 per cent of the finance required.

53

Table 4.4

Role of external assistance in Malian planning

Plan	(% of total finance)
1961-1965	56
1970-1972	86.4
1974-1978	88.9

Source: The Plans.

The results from the Recovery Programme (1970-1972) testify to the greater stability of internally generated resources as shown on Table 4.5. Whereas in the initial plan external sources were to finance 86.4 per cent of the entire programme, in practice this proportion was only 77.9 per cent. For internal sources realisations were 73.1 per cent of the revised plan while for external sources the proportion was only 46.6 per cent. When account is taken of inflation over the period it is most probably the case that external sources provided no more than one third of what was initially hoped.

Table 4.5

Financial results from the recovery programme
(MF millions)

	Internal sources (A)	External sources (B)	B/A%
Initial plan	10581	66993	86.4
Revised plan	17694	98074	84.7
Funds committed	15611	78024	83.3
Funds realised	12940	45730	77.9

Source: *Rapport d'Exécution du Programme de Redressement Économique et Financier 1970-1973;* Direction Générale du Plan et de la Statistique.

In the 1961-1965 plan it was proposed that the health sector would account for 2.1 per cent of total investment. The principal objectives were to construct and supply 63 dispensaries and to increase the number of hospital beds by 790. The plan also provided for a range of preventive measures with respect to the endemic diseases, extension of the PMI network, public hygiene and sanitary education. Thus even the first plan attached importance to preventive as well as curative health measures.

0.7 per cent of investment in the first plan was to be allocated to water and forestry. Unfortunately it is not possible to distinguish the water component. Nor is it possible to discuss the outcome of the plan since an ex post evaluation has not been carried out. In contrast, the Recovery Programme has been evaluated ex post and the details are

Table 4.6

Plans and outcomes in the recovery programme

	Initial plan	Revised plan	Funds committed	Funds realised
A Health				
(i) Planned				
Internal sources ⟩ (MF millions)	363	569	459	264
External sources ⟩	1651	3255	2166	637
Total	2014	3824	2625	901
% of all investments	2.6	3.3	2.8	1.5
(ii) Unplanned				
Internal sources ⟩ (MF millions)		44	44	44
External sources ⟩		1480	1481	1155
Total		1524	1525	1199
% of all investments		21	21.9	35.7
B Water				
(i) Planned				
Internal sources ⟩ (MF millions)			209	209
External sources ⟩	3288	3949	2893	1853
Total	3288	3949	3102	2062
% of all investments	4.2	3.4	3.3	3.4
(ii) Unplanned				
Internal sources ⟩ (MF millions)			23	23
External sources ⟩		260	260	
Total		260	283	23
% of all investments		3.6	4.1	0.7

Source: *Rapport d'Exécution du Programme de Redressement Économique et Financier 1970-1973;* Direction Generale du Plan et de la Statistique.

reported on Table 4.6. The table shows that while initially investment in health was to account for 2.6 per cent of the total, the final outcome was only 1.5 per cent, which was largely due to the failure of external aid, despite commitments of MF 2,166 millions. In fact, external aid disbursements for health were only 29 per cent of commitments, and 20 per cent of the figure in the revised plan. Relatively speaking the performance in regard to internal sources was less disappointing, realisations were only 46 per cent of the revised plan, while for internal sources as a whole performance was considerably better than this, as has already been pointed out (73.1 per cent). These observations suggest that relatively speaking the health sector has been a neglected area as far as the plan is concerned. However, for unplanned (hors plan) investment, the health sector has performed well with disbursements equal to 35.7 per cent of the total. Whereas in the revised planning stage unplanned investment in health was 40 per cent of planned investment, eventually the former surpassed the latter by 33 per cent. This suggests that the plan is not a useful guide to future investment in the health sector.

Five Year Plan 1974-1978

Like its predecessors the most recent plan lists a series of projects which Mali hopes to finance over the five year period. The projects associated with public health are described briefly in Appendix 1. Whereas for the plan as a whole it was intended that 88.9 per cent of investments would be financed externally, in the area of health the external financing factor is as high as 93 per cent. In view of what has been said earlier in relation to the unpredictability of external finance, it might be expected that especially as far as health is concerned, the plan was vulnerable ab initio.

Whereas in the first plan health accounted for 2.1 per cent of total investment and 2.6 per cent in the recovery programme, in the most recent plan health still only accounts for 2.5 per cent of total planned investment. Thus it can be said that at least as far as the plan is concerned, Mali has not attached any high priority to health and that its relative unimportance has been stable over a twenty year period. Table 4.7 records the planned investments in the various sectors. The table indicates that preventive health measures carry a relatively low weight in the plan, as do hygiene and sanitation. The categories included in Table 4.7 are intended loosely to cover expenditures in the delivery of 'basic needs', on which basis these items account for 12.4 per cent of the grand total. During the period of the plan it was intended to incur the following recurrent costs in MSP:

	MF millions
Personnel	11962.3
Material	9702.3
Total	21664.5

Source: *Plan Quinquennal,* p.390.

i.e., 55 per cent of these costs would be for personnel. These figures imply a gearing between investment and recurrent costs of 2.23 (i.e., 21664.5/9721.8).

Table 4.7
Allocation of investment in the Five Year Plan (1974-1978)

	MF millions (1974 prices)	Percentage of total investment
Public health	9721.8	2.5
Preventive	1436.9	0.4
Curative	8284.9	2.1
Social affairs	538.7	0.1
Education	24090.7	6.1
Primary	704.0	0.2
Secondary	3959.9	1.0
Higher	2927.0	0.7
Adult literacy	1989.4	0.5
Other	14510.4	3.7
Water	13877.2	3.5
Urban	5606.1	1.4
Rural	8271.1	2.1
Hygiene	775.0	0.2
		12.4
Sub-total	49003.4	
Grand total	395200.0	

Source: *Plan Quinquennal de Dévelopment Économique et Social 1974-1978;* Direction Generale du Plan et de la Statistique.

Progress with the plan

Since the period of the plan has yet to expire it is not possible to conduct an ex post evaluation of disbursement-commitment ratios as was done with the recovery programme. At the end of 1976 the initial investment estimates of MSP were revised upwards by 15 per cent reflecting inflation and project re-evaluation. Thus the investment costs of MSP rose from MF 9721.8 millions to MF 11180 millions. Table 4.8 records the status of this programme as of the end of 1976. Unfortunately the situation has changed little since this time, therefore the figures on Table 4.8 are still representative. Updated information may, however, be found in Appendix 1. While the disbursement ratio had reached 17 per cent as of the end of 1976, it is now probably no more than 20 per cent. The average disbursement ratio for the plan as a whole was 29 per cent, therefore it is evident that the investment activities of MSP have been laggard. However, in marked contrast the ratio for education was 35 per cent and for transportation and communications it was as high as 45 per cent. The disbursement ratio of MSP has been amongst the lowest and it seems likely that its relative performance will have deteriorated further since 1976.

Table 4.8

Progress with the Five Year Plan at MSP
as of 31 December 1976

	MF millions	% of revised planned investment
Disbursements	1896.8	17.0
Internal resources	259.0	
External resources	1637.8	
+ Commitments	2416.6	21.6
Internal resources	281.5	
External resources	2135.1	
+ Probable commitments	4821.4	43.1
+ Unplanned project commitments	7080.0	63.3

Source: *Actualisation et Situation des Projects d'Investissements de la Santé Publique au 31 December 1976;* March 1977, Ministère du Plan.

Another interesting feature of Table 4.8 is that while external resources were supposed to finance 93 per cent of MSP's investment programme only 86.3 per cent of disbursements have been financed externally. However, when commitments are added into the calculation this proportion rises to 88.4 per cent. This repeats the qualitative pattern that was observed in relation to the recovery programme (see Table 4.6) where external aid performance was relatively poor. It now seems that the estimates of probable commitments were far too optimistic in view of the lack of progress with MSP's part of the plan since 1976.

MF 2,258.6 millions of commitments for MSP projects outside the plan had accumulated by the end of 1976, 96.3 per cent of which were to be financed externally. However, only MF 501.5 millions, or 22.2 per cent of these had been disbursed. Since most of these projects bear a relation to those included in the plan, it could be claimed that 63.3 per cent of planned investment might be achieved. On this basis, a more realistic estimate of the disbursement ratio would be about 26 per cent.

Health and basic needs in the State Budget

Proportionately speaking the MSP budget has been declining over the past decade as is indicated by Table 4.9.

Table 4.9

Percentage share of health in the State Budget

Year	% Share
1965	10.6
1973	10.1
1974	9.9
1975	9.2
1976	8.2
1977	7.4
1978	7.3

Source: *Budget d'État*, *Recaputulation Generale;* Direction Nationale du Budget.

Indeed, between 1973 and 1977 there was a considerable deceleration in the percentage allocation to MSP. Table 4.10 conveys revealed budgetary priorities and indicates that since 1973 education and health in particular have been losing ground to defence expenditures. Table 4.10 also shows that since 1973 the proportion of the budget that has been allocated for personnel declined slightly from 83.3 per cent. The allocation of expenditures for water supply has continued to remain derisory, and out of all proportion to the role of water in Mali's socioeconomic development. About half of one per cent of the budget is allocated for such purposes.

Yet relatively speaking Malian per capita health expenditures through the State Budget are high, as evidenced by Table 4.11. Out of the African countries listed on this table, Mali's budgetary allocation is second only to Malawi's, although of course Mali's per capita expenditure on health remains below the average of $2.21. This is due to Mali's low per capita income status. However, relative to its per capita income, a regression analysis indicates that Mali's per capita expenditures on health through the budget are 56 per cent higher than the norm. [13] Thus Mali's budgetary income allocation for MSP remains the highest in Africa when adjusting for income status. But if the trend in Table 4.9 continues this position could easily be undermined.

Naturally, great care should be taken in making such comparisons, since the coverage of different budgetary aggregates is likely to diverge quite markedly from country to country. Also, what matters is the total resource allocation for health, private as well as public, and reference has

Table 4.10

Allocation of State Budget (MF millions)

Ministry	1973	1977	1978
Foreign affairs	731.6	1425.1	1750.8
% of State Budget	2.6	2.5	2.8
Defence	4900.3	12643.3	13966.6
% of State Budget	17.4	22.4	22.7
Finance and commerce	1171.3	1931.7	2026.1
% of State Budget	4.2	3.4	3.3
Water and energy	92.5	272.4	272.6
% of State Budget	0.3	0.5	0.4
Industrial development and tourism	na	113.1	94.8
% of State Budget		0.2	0.1
Transport and public works	na	1059.4	1168.3
% of State Budget		1.9	1.9
Rural development	na	1943.5	2303.5
% of State Budget		3.4	3.7
Education	9034.7	15198.5	17310.2
% of State Budget	32.1	26.9	28.1
Youth, sports and culture	152.0	457.4	574.2
% of State Budget	0.5	0.8	0.9
Health	2861.1	4171.4	4518.0
% of State Budget	10.1	7.4	7.3
Social affairs	187.0	328.6	365.2
% of State Budget	0.7	0.6	0.6
Total State Budget	28134.9	56387.6	61488.6
Personnel	23437.3	44109.2	48904.9
%	83.3	78.2	79.5
Material	4697.6	12278.4	12583.7
%	16.7	21.8	20.5

Source: *Budget d'État, Recapitulation Générale 1974, 1978;*
Direction Nationale du Budget.

Table 4.11

Budget and per capita health expenditures
selected African countries (1975)

Country	Health as % of total budget	Per capita expend on health $
Mali	9.2	1.70
Botswana	2.9	.33
Cameroon	2.3	.01
Central African Empire	5.3	.01
Ethiopia	5.4	1.31
Gabon	1.6	11.30
Ghana	8.5	8.29
Ivory Coast	6.9	.01
Lesotho	8.1	1.75
Liberia	3.7	2.88
Madagascar	4.4	1.31
Malawi	11.1	2.58
Niger	6.5	1.09
Nigeria	2.0	.99
Sierra Leone	5.7	1.42
Somalia	6.6	1.51
Sudan	2.2	1.01
Swaziland	7.6	4.83
Tanzania	5.8	2.74
Uganda	6.2	1.78
Upper Volta	8.1	.78
Zaire	2.7	1.20
Average	5.57	2.21

Source: Computed from *Europa Yearbook, A World Survey* (London: Europa Publishers, 1977).

already been made to the fact that in Mali private health expenditures, especially on drugs, are large relative to public expenditure on health. Furthermore, it is critical to take into account the distribution of these expenditures among the population. Since the vast majority of health services cease at the cercle level and since 32 per cent of the population live in the urban areas and the central arrondissement of each cercle, it may be argued that roughly speaking no more than 32 per cent of the population directly benefit from these expenditures, with the greater emphasis on the urban areas (at least in financial terms). However, if it is further assumed that the catchment area of a rural dispensary is the arrondissement itself, it follows that approximately another 23 per cent

Table 4.12

Allocation of National Budget—Ministère de la Santé Publique (MF millions)

	Personnel			Material			Total		
	1973	1977	1978	1973	1977	1978	1973	1977	1978
Central administration	97.5	196.2	197.3	4.3	13.5	14.2	101.8	209.7	211.5
% of MSP budget							4.5	6.4	6.0
Hospitals and med-care	473.8	828.0	932.8	(Food) 189.7	(Food) 217.11 (Other) 85.3	(Food) 226.6 (Other) 91.3	663.5	1130.4	1250.7
% of MSP budget							29.5	34.3	35.2
Training of nurses and midwives	81.2	127.4	149.8	34.8	31.0	32.5	116.0	158.4	182.3
% of MSP budget							5.2	4.8	5.1
PMI	51.0	81.7	94.8	1.4	5.4	5.7	52.4	87.1	100.5
% of MSP budget							2.3	2.6	2.8
Nutrition division	5.0	5.5	6.6	2.0	4.3	4.5	7.0	9.8	11.1
% of MSP budget							0.3	0.3	0.3
Service des Grandes Endémies	133.8	168.2	185.1	10.3	12.0	12.6	141.1	180.2	197.7
% of MSP budget							6.3	5.5	5.6
Other socio-preventive medicine	61.1	113.6	132.3	16.1	24.2	25.7	77.2	137.8	158.0
% of MSP budget							3.4	4.2	4.4
Public hygiene	46.6	69.5	77.9	3.1	16.9	17.7	49.7	86.4	95.6
% of MSP budget							2.2	2.6	2.7
Lutte anti TB	34.1	45.7	58.7	10.9	16.7	17.5	45.0	62.4	76.2
% of MSP budget							2.0	1.9	2.1
Ph. d'Appro	33.8	43.4	50.2	(Drugs) 814.9 (Other) 1.6	(Drugs) 1000.0 (Other) 5.0	(Drugs) 1050.0 (Other) 5.2	850.3	1048.4	1105.4
% of MSP budget							37.8	31.8	31.1
Other	67.3	137.0	114.5	72.4	47.7	49.5	139.2	185.7	164.0
% of MSP budget							6.2	5.6	4.6
Total	1085.2	1816.2	2000.0	1161.5	1479.1	1553.0	2246.7	3295.3	3553.0
% of total budget	5.9	5.6	5.4	20.9	13.9	13.8	9.3	6.6	6.5

Source: *Budget d'État; Recaputulation Génerale 1974, 1978; Direction Nationale du Budget*

of the population will benefit from the more limited services of these dispensaries, making a total of 55 per cent of the population who benefit in one way or another from the MSP's expenditures through the State Budget.

The National Budget

Table 4.12 summarises the allocation of MSP's expenditures in the National Budget and indicates that since 1973, expenditures on hospitals and medical care have increased from 29.3 per cent of the MSP budget to 35.2 per cent. This increase has largely reflected higher expenditures on personnel which in turn have reflected the growth in the number of doctors. Nevertheless, MSP's share in the total personnel budget has declined slightly from 5.9 per cent in 1973 to 5.4 per cent in 1978.

Over the same period the share of expenditures of the Pharmacie d' Approvisionnement declined from 37.8 per cent to 31.1 per cent reflecting an average annual rate of growth for drug expenditures of 5.2 per cent in money terms—a rate of growth which is unlikely to have kept up with the rate of drug price inflation. On the other hand, attempts to bring cheaper drugs might have reversed this trend. Another activity which lost ground over the period was the Service des Grandes Endemies, falling back from 6.3 per cent in 1973 to 5.6 per cent in 1978. However, the proportion of expenditures on the Lutte Anti-TB remained stable as did the allocation for training, while expenditures on PMI grew from 2.3 per cent to 2.8 per cent.

Table 4.13

Percentage of National Budget allocated
to preventative and curative medicine
(%)

	1973	1977	1978
Curative*	78.7	76.5	76.0
Preventive	16.8	17.1	18.0
Central administrative	4.5	6.4	6.0

*'Curative' includes 'hospitals + medical care', 'training of nurses and midwives', 'Pharmacie d'Approvisionnement' and 'other' from Table 4.12.

Table 4.13 attempts to determine the balance of MSP's expenditures between preventive and curative medicine and is derived from Table 4.12. The table indicates that the balance of expenditures has been moving in favour of preventive medicine at the expense of curative medicine, but that the allocation of expenditures to preventive medicine has been relatively low. It will be recalled that in the latest five year plan preventive medicine was to account for 14.8 per cent of MSP's investment expenditures. It should also be recalled that these developments have occurred against a back-drop of a declining importance of MSP expenditures in the budget. Indeed, whereas between 1975-1977 the annual rate of growth of government employment was as high as 5.0 per cent, the rate of growth of MSP employment was only 1.2 per cent.

The budgetary figures to which reference has been made so far are for the revised proposals (with the exception of 1978). However, certain proposals may not be implemented for various administrative and practical reasons, and Table 4.14 summarises the disbursement factor for the MSP budget in relation to the revised proposals and eventual commitments. The table shows that for the most part, commitments bear a strong relationship with the revised proposals, and that the disbursement ratio tends to be very high. The exception of 1976 reflects a very low disbursement ratio for expenditures on materials; the disbursement ratio for personnel expenditures remained high. Therefore, it is the exception rather than the rule that disbursement ratios are low.

Table 4.14

Disbursement factors in MSP budget (%)

	1974	1975	1976	1977
Relative to:				
Proposals	98.5	98.5	65.7	98.4
· Commitments	98.8	99.1	97.9	98.6

Source: Direction Nationale du Budget.

Table 4.15 draws attention to the fact that the vast majority of budgetary expenditures are for recurrent costs rather than investment. Indeed, the pattern with MSP as with other departments is for investment to be financed by external aid while operating costs and maintenance are financial out of internal budgetary resources. Therefore the task of the budget is to ensure that these investments remain functional. All the investment accrues through the National Budget; the Regional Budget is devoted entirely to operating costs. The table indicates that the budgetary allocation for investment is extremely low and that in recent years it has been halved. Moreover, it should be pointed out that in many respects the distinction between investment and operating costs is blurred. For example, substantial repairs to buildings tend to be considered as investment. Therefore, new capital formation is considerably lower than the figures presented in Table 4.15.

Table 4.15

Investment expenditures in MSP budget

	1976	1977	1978
MF millions	82.5	52.0	44.2
% of State budget	2.0	1.2	1.0

Source: CAF de Ministère de la Santé Publique.

Regional Budget

The relationship between the Regional and State Budgets has already been described, and in terms of expenditures the Regional Budget is relatively unimportant as can be seen from Table 4.16. In fact the Retional Budget has been declining in importance as far as total expenditures are concerned, although the importance of the regional health budget has been stable. Also, roughly one-fifth of health expenditures accrue through the Regional Budget while only one-tenth of total expenditures accrue in this way. Therefore, for health expenditures the Regional Budget continues to be an important institution.

Table 4.16

Shares in State Budget (%)

Health:					
Regional Budget	21.9	21.3	21.3	21.0	21.4
National Budget	78.1	78.7	78.7	79.0	78.6
Total:					
Regional Budget	15.3	13.9	13.3	11.6	10.9
National Budget	84.7	86.1	86.7	88.4	89.1

Source: Direction Nationale du Budget.

Table 4.17 summarises the allocation of the Regional Budget in terms of per capita expenditure by region. The table draws attention to a strong bias in favour of the second region which most probably reflects the presence of the capital. It also draws attention to the unfavourable distribution of the fifth region where the people of Mopti receive 40 per cent of their counterparts in Bamako. However, since national budgetary expenditures have a regional dimension too, a more reliable analysis of the fiscal distribution would have to take these into consideration. Nevertheless, it is probable that the indications of Table 4.17 would be reflected in such a broader investigation.

Table 4.17

Per capita expenditure in the Regional Budget (MF)

	1973	1977	1978
Kayes	760	1110	1109
Bamako	786	1342	1496
Sikasso	506	837	823
Segou	611	860	925
Mopti	550	701	599
Gao	925	1059	1104
Total	673	983	1008

Based in provisional results from the 1976 census.

Source: *Budget d'État, Recapitulation Générale 1974, 1978;*
          Direction Nationale du Budget.

Table 4.18 summarises the allocation of the Regional Budget in terms of health-related expenditures. The most important element in the regions' expenditures is education, while expenditures on AM constitute an important allocation for all regions except the second. The allocation for rural water supply is consistently negligible across all of the regions as is also the case for the Service d'Hygiene and the PMI. Thus preventive health plays an even lower role in the Regional Budget than it does in the National Budget.

Table 4.18

Allocations of Regional Budget (MF millions)

	Personnel			Material			Total		
	1973	1977	1978	1973	1977	1978	1973	1977	1978
Kayes									
Service d'Hygiene	3.7	2.9	5.2	0.2	0.3	0.3	3.9	3.2	5.5
% of Regional Budget							0.6	0.3	0.6
PMI	2.6	3.3	1.7	0.2	0.3	0.3	2.8	3.6	2.0
% of Regional Budget							0.4	0.4	0.2
Assistance Médicale	97.4	116.5	131.9	1.4	4.0	5.2	98.8	120.5	137.1
% of Regional Budget							14.9	12.5	14.2
Education	427.2	662.3	629.2	13.0	16.9	16.7	440.2	679.2	645.9
% of Regional Budget							66.5	70.2	66.8
Rural water supply	n/a	–	–	0.2	0.4	0.4	n/a	0.4	0.4
% of Regional Budget							n/a	0.0	0.0
Bamako									
Service d'Hygiene	–	–	–	0.4	–	–	0.4	–	–
% of Regional Budget							0.0		
PMI	–	–	–	0.6	–	–	0.6	–	–
% of Regional Budget							0.1		
Assistance Médicale	155.6	14.7	23.5	5.0	4.9	5.2	160.6	19.6	28.7
% of Regional Budget							15.5	1.1	1.5
Education	699.6	1228.4	1398.8	38.0	50.2	52.7	737.6	1278.6	1451.5
% of Regional Budget							71.1	72.2	73.5
Rural water supply	4.7	6.0	–	1.1	2.0	2.1	5.8	8.0	2.1
% of Regional Budget							0.6	0.5	0.1
Sikasso									
Service d'Hygiene	2.0	3.8	3.0	0.2	0.3	0.3	2.2	4.1	3.3
% of Regional Budget							0.4	0.4	0.3
PMI	4.0	6.0	6.8	0.5	0.5	0.5	4.5	6.5	7.3
% of Regional Budget							0.8	0.7	0.8
Assistance Médicale	86.5	132.7	143.1	4.3	4.4	4.6	90.8	137.1	147.7
% of Regional Budget							15.3	14.0	15.3
Education	354.0	635.4	589.7	8.5	8.5	8.9	362.5	643.9	598.8
% of Regional Budget							61.1	65.6	62.1
Rural water supply	n/a	–	–	n/a	–	–	n/a	–	–
% of Regional Budget							n/a	–	–

Table 4.18 (continued)

	Personnel			Material			Total		
	1973	1977	1978	1973	1977	1978	1973	1977	1978
Segou									
Service d'Hygiene	3.2	6.3	5.8	2.1	1.1	1.1	6.7	7.4	6.9
% of Regional Budget							1.1	0.9	0.8
PMI	1.4	1.7	2.6		1.0	1.1		2.7	3.7
% of Regional Budget								0.3	0.4
Assistance Médicale	70.5	108.0	120.6	4.4	5.2	5.5	74.9	110.2	126.1
% of Regional Budget							12.5	13.0	13.8
Education	361.6	523.4	560.7	16.6	17.2	20.1	378.2	540.6	580.8
% of Regional Budget							62.9	63.9	63.8
Rural water supply	1.3	4.4	4.9	0.2	0.4	0.4	1.5	4.8	5.3
% of Regional Budget							0.2	0.6	0.6
Mopti									
Service d'Hygiene	2.5	4.7	4.0	0.5	0.7	0.7	3.0	5.4	4.7
% of Regional Budget							0.4	0.6	0.6
PMI	2.1	4.3	4.0	0.2	0.4	0.4	2.3	4.7	4.4
% of Regional Budget							0.3	0.5	0.6
Assistance Médicale	104.1	145.6	159.4	7.6	8.6	9.0	111.8	154.2	168.4
% of Regional Budget							16.5	17.8	22.7
Education	375.8	496.3	330.3	9.4	25.6	26.7	385.2	521.9	357.0
% of Regional Budget							56.7	60.2	48.0
Rural water supply	7.1	9.9	11.1	0.8	5.1	5.4	7.9	15.0	16.5
% of Regional Budget							1.2	1.7	2.2
Gao									
Service d'Hygiene	–	–	–	0.3	0.3	0.4	0.3	0.3	0.4
% of Regional Budget							0.0	0.0	0.1
PMI	–	–	–	0.5	0.6	0.6	0.5	0.6	0.6
% of Regional Budget							0.1	0.1	0.1
Assistance Médicale	78.7	104.2	115.5	4.1	4.5	4.7	82.8	108.7	120.2
% of Regional Budget							12.4	14.2	15.0
Education	421.0	466.7	479.9	12.8	14.1	14.8	433.8	480.8	494.7
% of Regional Budget							64.8	62.7	61.9
Rural water supply	19.3	3.4	2.6	0.3	0.3	0.3	19.6	3.7	2.9
% of Regional Budget							2.9	0.5	0.4

Source: *Budget d'État, Recapitulation Générale 1974, 1978;* Direction Nationale du Budget.

External assistance

As has already been described, external assistance was ascribed a pre-
dominant role in Mali's investment plan. Indeed, most probably more
than 90 per cent of capital formation is financed by external assistance
and Table 4.19 indicates that external assistance has tended to surpass
capital formation by a substantial margin, implying that external finance
has been used to pay for operating costs. However, tax revenue has been
growing relative to external assistance and in 1978 was expected that
external assistance would be about 8 per cent of the State Budget.

Table 4.19

Structure of State Budget (MF millions)

	1974	1975	1976	1977	1978
Expenditure					
Current	31100	37300	44500	52000	57200
Capital	500	1600	2300	3000	4300
Financing					
Revenue	24000	28800	36700	46000	56500
External	6600	11500	5400	5000	5000
Other internal	1000	- 1400	4700	4000	0

Source: Data provided by Malian authorities

Unfortunately, there are no comprehensive data on the disbursement
of external assistance in relation to health and associated fields. Indeed,
the fact that the authorities could not provide such comprehensive doc-
umentation must be a matter for concern since it suggests that there is
little co-ordination and planning in the absorbtion of external assistance.
Nevertheless, Table 4.20 attempts to assemble the available information
on external assistance in the fields of health and related areas. The data
provided are an amalgam of commitments and disbursements and the
coverage has been necessarily selective. It is also incomplete since there
are numerous religious and secular missions in the country that are involved in health, training, well-drilling, etc. It would be virtually impossible to document their activities and to estimate the resource transfer
that is involved, but it is most probably large—running into the millions
of dollars. However, these resources are a direct transfer to the people
and do not accrue via the State Budget. In addition to these sources are
the remittances in kind of Malians working overseas. There are numerous
instances where relatives abroad had sent drugs to their villages in Mali
and where 'sister towns' in France had contributed to various health-
related activities. For example in Koutiola the people of Alençon were
contributing to the construction of an X-ray block.

Table 4.20

External assistance

Project	Donor	Commitment US$	Duration	Type of assistance
Health.				
Assistance to health services	WHO	182800	1977	Epidemiologist, sanitation engineer, nurse, technical operator.
Development of family planning programme	UNFPA/WHO	1096085	1975-9	Community development, family planning, primary health care.
Health programme	UNICEF	72000	1976-7	PMI.
Nutrition assistance	WFP	285071	1977	Assistance to ten hospitals.
Training personnel	WHO	104000	1977	Bursaries and courses.
Supervising nurses	WHO	37600	1977	
Medical assistance	WHO	13000	1977	Subvention and material.
Rural health	USAID	3890000	1977-80	Pilot scheme at Yelimane and Koro.
Medical team	China	n/a	1977	40 people at Sikasso, Kati and Makola.
Hospital assistance	USSR	n/a	1977	Material, drugs, 26 doctors at Bamako, Kayes, Gao, Mopti.
Study for hygiene centre	Italy	11000	1977	At Niafunké.
Dispensary	CIMADE	90000	1974-7	At Doila, construction and equipment.
Nat. Inst. for traditional medicine	CUOS	36547	1977-8	To develop traditional remedies.
Dispensary repairs	Int'l plan	23000	1977	At Banamba.
Pharmaceuticals	CARE	28000	1976-7	Gift to MSP.
Health service	CNAPVS	219400	1974-5	Reinforcement since the drought.
Grandes Endémies	UNICEF	34000	1974	
Sepau	UNICEF	49000	1974-6	Construction of stores, garages and antennae.
Project CSM	UNICEF	10600	1974-6	Nutrition programme.
Grandes Endémies	FFRF	58500	1974-7	For bicycles, mobylettes, offices, etc.
Hospital services	FFRF	85800	1974-7	Operating blocks and general construction at Dire.
Medical care	Fonds Chessom	40400	1975	Assistance at Pt. 'C' and AM at Koulikoro.
Health services	S. Arabia	4790000	1975-7	Drugs, equipment, dental centres.
Pediatric centre	Red Cross	64715	1975-6	Construction at Tombouctou.
Nutrition programme	CIMADE	10600	1977	Centre at Goundam.
Health services	Switzerland	n/a	1978-80	Wells, surgery, drugs, mobylettes in Sikasso region.

Table 4.20 (continued)

Project	Donor	Commitment US$	Duration	Type of assistance
Water				
Water supply	W. Germany	7900000	1977-81	Kita
Underground water	UNDP/BTC	5812568	1977-81	Research and evaluation
Water supply	UNCDF	1429000	1976-8	Nioro in collaboration with FAC.
Underground water	UNICEF	1651000	1977-81	Purchase of material
Water supply	FED	3497500	1974-7	Studies for Mopti, Sévaré and Nara.
Water supply	CEAO	109000	1977	Studies at Gao, Markala, Kayes and Bougouni.
Water supply	FAC	500000	1977-8	Nioro in collaboration with UNCDF.
Wells	FAC	550000	1974-7	Gao.
Water supply	FAC	220000	1975-7	Study at Koutiala.
Drilling	USSR	n/a	1976-7	4 experts at Kulano and Kita.
Urban water	Italy	235000	1976	Studies at Nioro, Dia, Niafunké, Bankass and Koro.
Water supply	UK	1020000	1976-7	Sikasso.
Wells	AFRICARE	121000	1975-8	Tombouctou, Goundam and Banamba.
Equipment	CIMADE	100000	1973	Bankass.
Education				
Education programme	UNICEF	100000	1976-7	Ruralisation of basic education.
Literacy	USSR	n/a	1976-9	Construction and equipment for National Centre at Bamako in collaboration with UNICEF.
Classes	CARE	139000	1976	Construction in the second region.
Literacy	Euro action Sahel	34250	1977-8	In Songhi and Tamacheq.
Literacy	ACDI	2206000	1975-8	Functional literacy in the cotton zone.
Food				
	FED	n/a	1977	500 tonnes of powdered milk, 112 tonnes of butter.
	W. Germany	980000	1977	Purchase of cereals.

Source: Rapport sur les Assistances Extérieres en Matière de Développement, UNDP, Mali 1977; CAF, Ministère de la Santé Publique.

Key: CIMADE Protestant organisation (Paris)
CUOS Canadian Universities Overseas Service
FFRF Fondation Françaises Raoul Follereau
UNCDF UN Capital Development Fund
CEAD Commounauté Économique de l'Afrique Ouest
ACDI Agence Canadienne de Développement International

Policy issues in resource allocation

It should be recalled at the outset that to improve health it may not be necessary to intervene in the health sector directly as is argued in Chapter 3. Improvements to productivity, especially of the poor, will most probably improve nutritional status which in turn will tend to improve health status. In general, however, it will be necessary to intervene on a multi-disciplinary basis by combining preventive and curative health measures (see Appendix 2) as well as to co-ordinate the health benefits, direct and indirect, that might be associated with interventions with regard to education, water supply, sanitation, etc., and of course medical care itself. As described in Chapter 3, it will be necessary for health planners to take into consideration the impact and delivery linkages associated with the various basic needs interventions in order to attain the greatest possible improvements in health status for given availabilities of human and pecuniary resources.

Before entering into a discussion of how in the Malian context such a basic needs approach to health policy might be applied and how existing resources might be more effectively used in relation to health status, it is necessary to consider a number of characteristics of Mali's resource mobilisation with respect to health.

Recurrent costs, investment and aid

In principle there should be a relationship between recurrent cost expenditures and the stock of capital equipment. As the stock of schools, clinics, etc., increases more recurrent expenditures on teachers' salaries, drugs, etc., will be required. More Land Rovers require more gas and spare parts to run them. Recurrent cost requirements will vary from activity to activity. Up to a point higher development costs may be incurred in order to lower the associated recurrent cost expenditures, drawing attention to the arbitrary distinction between the two kinds of expenditures as far as the project as a whole is concerned.

As has already been explained, in Mali there is a division of labour between the resource mobilisation for recurrent and development expenditures. The Malians through the State Budget take care of the former while foreign assistance is responsible for the latter. In addition the Regional Budget is responsible for recurrent expenditures that service the capital that has been installed through the National Budget and external assistance.

It is most probably the case that the list of projects in the five year plan is heavily influenced by where the authorities consider external donors will be interested. In the health sector, although the Malians have certain broad priorities in regard to preventive health, it appears that investment follows the interests of the external donors both in terms of volume and focus. By and large the donors do not wish to be involved in recurrent expenditures, so it is left to the Malians to find these resources. Instead of figuring what volume of investment they can afford to service with a recurrent budget, development and recurrent expenditures have not been well planned, with the result that much of the development expenditures is either under-productive or not productive at all. Thus there are school buildings without teachers, dispensaries without drugs, vehicles without gas and spare parts, hospital equipment without essential inputs, etc., etc.

Foreign aid appears to be free to the Malians and this no doubt accounts for a certain lack of discrimination in the planning of externally financed development expenditure. If it costs nothing why turn offers down? Apart from leading to a misallocation of external resources on a global basis, in practice foreign aid may not be free to the Malians. First, externally financed projects tie up scarce man-power which may be more carefully applied to activities other than receiving foreign missions and administering to their projects. Secondly, externally financed developments tie up a limited recurrent cost budget; in allocating recurrent resources to 'free' projects the functioning of other projects may begin to suffer. In the health and related sectors there are no glaring examples of outlandish projects such as ultra modern hospitals which sap large proportions of the budget at the expense of more productive activities. Nevertheless, it is evident that this problem exists on a less dramatic scale in Mali.

It must therefore be asked whether future development aid as presently conceived is appropriate in Mali. There is little point in supplying Land Rovers if they run a high risk of being immobilised after a short while. The negative reaction is to withhold aid until the Malians ensure that they can meet the associated recurrent costs. Certainly any project involvement by the Malians or any other institutio. should require careful scrutiny of its recurrent cost implications as a precondition. Alternatively, higher development costs might be incurred in order to save on future recurrent expenditures; but this may not be in the broader development interests of the country.

The positive reaction would be to consider recurrent expenditures as investment which both in principle and practice are no different to the investment that takes place through so-called development expenditures. The gasoline that puts the Land Rovers back on the road, the spare parts that put hospital equipment back into service, the drugs that are essential to the functioning of the dispensaries, etc., have high rates of return in Mali and while they are recurrent expenditures it would be more appropriate to consider them as legitimate investment expenditures. Investment should therefore be broken down into its development and recurrent components. In Mali, it is evident that greater emphasis is required on the recurrent component, yet external donors have so far shunned involvement in this area at the expense of themselves as well as the intended beneficiaries. It would therefore be more appropriate for donors to consider investment as a whole rather than preoccupying themselves exclusively with the development component, and cost benefit calculations should be based on the totality of investment, development as well as recurrent. The negative reaction of insisting that the Malians guarantee the provision of the recurrent component until the development component is provided is neither sound development economics, nor is it appropriate to the broader role that the donors play.

This requires greater donor co-operation for several reasons. First, there is no co-ordination within MSP in relation to foreign assistance in the health sector. Projects seem to be tabled haphazardly and it is only by chance that donors discover what other donors are doing in what may be closely related activities. Secondly, in order to invoke a positive response to the recurrent cost problem donor co-ordination will most probably be necessary. Thirdly, it is evident that the number of foreign donors is expanding. What used to be regarded as a French area of influence now enjoys the assistance of a number of other European countries, the US, China, the USSR and Saudi Arabia. The need for donor co-ordination has grown considerably in recent years.

Policy choices

As has been pointed out, about 7 per cent of the State Budget is allocated to MSP and the allocation has been steadily declining. If indeed more effective resources are to be mobilised for health and related purposes a number of policy options may be considered.

(i) Focus budgetary growth on health and related activities.
(ii) Re-allocate the existing budget.
(iii) Re-allocate the existing health budget.
(iv) Review consumer-charging policies.
(v) Decentralise present budgetary institutions.

These and other policy options should not of course be considered separately; it is possible to proceed on all fronts at the same time.

(i) The focus of budgetary growth:

Table 4.21 summarises tax revenue in Mali and its composition. By far the most important revenue source are the taxes on international trade which have the undesirable effects of distorting the pattern of Mali's trade. In 1975-6 the authorities made a concerted effort to

74

increase the tax-take, yet because of GDP growth this only raised the ratio of tax revenue to GDP to 12.1 per cent. Table 4.22 provided for purposes of comparing this ratio with similar ratios in other countries in order to judge whether it is reasonable to expect the fiscal authorities in Mali to raise additional revenue. Relative to other African countries the revenue:GDP ratio in Mali is low,* especially for a political economy which in practice is socialistic. If say Mali were to raise this ratio by five percentage points revenue would grow by about MF 17,500 millions which would easily accommodate any expansion in the MSP budget.

Table 4.21

Tax revenue and GDP (MF millions)

	1973	1974	1975	1976
Tax revenue	21214	22960	27736	34967
Income and profits	2392	4256	3924	6437
Indirect	2795	2308	3614	3859
Poll tax	3043	3128	3552	3919
Customs and Excise	8139	9046	11195	12180
Export taxes	1515	1210	861	1950
Livestock	—	—	929	961
Revenue ÷ GDP (%)	11.6	11.7	10.7	12.1

Source: Malian authorities for tax data.

Table 4.22

Government revenue as a percentage of GDP in 1973

Algeria	38.3	The Gambia	20.1	Nigeria	17.2
Benin	15.7	Chana	11.7	Senegal	13.3
Burundi	11.3	Guinea	18.6	Sierra Leone	16.3
Camaroon	17.3	Ivory Coast	21.2	Somalia	27.5
CAE	20.4	Liberia	16.9	Sudan	31.6
Chad	14.4	Mauritania	17.1	Togo	13.9
Congo	22.4	Morocco	19.1	Upper Volta	11.7
Gabon	21.9	Niger	11.4		

Source: *World Tables 1976,* page 442, World Bank.

However, more important than average tax rates is the structure of marginal tax rates since these will determine the structure of incentives. The critical problem is whether the disincentive effects of higher tax

*Based on a regression for 32 African countries between the revenue: GDP ratio and GDP per capita, the expected value of Mali's revenue ratio was calculated to be 18.53 per cent.

rates would be significant. It is known for example that the government's recent attempts to improve tax harvesting especially with respect to firms has caused a wave of bankruptcies. It is also noted that several of Mali's neighbours have similar revenue: GDP ratios. Clearly this is not the occasion for a comprehensive review of Mali's fiscal structure. However, a superficial reading suggests that the possibilities of additional revenue raising are worth exploring.

(ii) Re-allocating the State Budget:

Despite pressures to the contrary the Malian authorities have done well to limit the proportion of the State budget that is allocated for salaries, as may be seen from Table 4.23. Nevertheless, it is clear that what previously has been described as the political economy of the salariat is a major drain on budgetary resources. The issue is whether in future it is possible to limit further this resource expenditure and to allocate some of the balance to the health sector. This, of course, is a major political issue which the government has confronted in the past but without any real success. The government should be encouraged to continue its policy of expanding the budget for materials at the expense of personnel, however, it is as yet too early to judge whether the authorities have been succeeding in this regard.

Table 4.23

Percentage of State Budget: personnel

1974	1975	1976	1977	1978
83	80.3	83	78.2	79.5

Source: Direction Nationale du Budget.

Table 4.10 has already summarised the allocation of the budget. In view of the importance attached to health as a productive sector it is essential that at the very least the declining share of MSP in the budget be stopped and that it should even be reversed. In this context an interim objective might be to aim for a 10 per cent allocation in future budgets. Indeed, this would be a measure of the importance that the government attaches to health as a productive sector. It is also important to increase the allocation of the budget for water and sanitation in view of the importance that these activities play in regard to public health. To trim about 5 per cent off the rest of the budget to favour these sectors should be feasible. Indeed, much of this could be taken up by budgetary growth so that real expenditures elsewhere need not be cut back. Since 1974 the budget has expanded at an average annual rate of 18 per cent of which about half may be attributed to inflation.

If (using 1978 as a base) the State Budget grows at 9 per cent per annum in real terms this will add MF 5534 millions in relation to a total health budget of MF 4518 millions in 1978. If, for illustrative purposes all of this increase were allocated to MSP, the MSP share in the 1979 budget would rise from 7.3 per cent to 15 per cent. Thus a 10 per cent target allocation for 1980 may even be conservative.

(iii) Re-allocating the health budget:

The allocation of the health budget has already been summarised in Tables 4.12 and 4.18. In this context the objective should be to strike an appropriate balance between preventive and curative health as explained in Appendix 2 and to integrate policies with respect to the delivery of basic needs as outlined in Chapter 3. Whatever the outcome of such an exercise it seems likely that the present health budget reflects a gross imbalance between its preventive and curative components. Both in the plan and in the budget, preventive health is of dimmunitive importance despite the government's progressive policy pronouncements to the contrary. However, attention is drawn to the fact (see Table 4.13) that proportionate expenditure on preventive measures has been increasing, but the pace has been slow. An interim objective might be to consolidate this progress and to raise the allocation to preventive measures from its current level of 18 per cent to 25 per cent by the early 1980s. In this context it should be recalled that expenditure on water provision and sanitation constitute preventive measures too, but these do not come under the MSP budget.

18.1 per cent of the hospitals and medical care budget—or 6.4 per cent of MSP's National budget—(see Table 4.12) is allocated for food. Since patients would in any event have had to pay for their food it seems reasonable to expect that patients bring their own food or they should pay for it while they are in hospital. If the food budget is eliminated and the balance is transferred to preventive health, this measure alone could raise the budgetary allocation to the suggested 25 per cent target.

Of the growth areas in the MSP budget it is encouraging to note the emphasis placed on PMI and public hygiene. But to realise a 25 per cent target, growth in these areas would have to be much stronger. In 1978 the growth in hospital expenditures was more than the total expenditure on either PMI or public hygiene.

(iv) Charge policy:

While government policy is for free health services, the fact remains that many services are paid for on either official or unofficial bases. The Malians themselves are traditionally used to paying for their cures;

it has been long standing practice to pay local healers for their services as well as traditional midwives. Therefore the basis exists for introducing a policy of payment where appropriate.

In the area of public health, however, there are numerous externalities since people tend to infect each other either directly or indirectly. Thus up to a point, it may be in the social interest to subsidise health services since the social benefit may be greater than the private benefit. In this context it would be desirable, for example, to distinguish between drugs which will prevent possible later contamination and which subsequently have a social externality from those such as aspirin, which do not. The same principle may be applied to other areas of the health sector. For example, while the costs of well construction and maintenance are high, the social benefits could be very large.

At the present time the following services are paid for:

drugs from the Pharmacie Populaire: at cost;
rural maternities: MF 300 per confinement;
urban maternities: MF 1000 per confinement;
hospitals: MF 200 per day.

Most probably all these rates reflect costs, to some degree although as has already been pointed out it is necessary to supplement the salaries of the rural matronnes with revenues from FGR drug sales. In addition, taxes and import duties mean that the public pay more than the true (private) cost of the drugs they buy from the Pharmacie Populaire. The Pharmacie Populaire has proposed that in order to reduce drug prices, drugs be exempted from import duties, a proposal which is unlikely to be popular with the Ministry of Finance. In any event it is important to distinguish between essential and inessential drugs and it should be possible to devise a tax structure that encourages the consumption of essential drugs while placing the burden of taxation on the inessential drugs along the principles set out in Appendix 3. Insofar as the essential drugs also have the social externalities previously described while the inessential drugs were purchased out of ignorance concerning their medical value, such a discriminatory tax policy would be socially beneficial from many points of view. In Mali these conditions are most probably fulfilled and the authorities should be encouraged to investigate such a policy as a component of a more comprehensive review of drug policy.

The services which are free are:

visits to AM;
visits to rural dispensaries;
drugs from the Pharmacie d'Approvisionnement;
visits to PMI;
Services des Grandes Endémies;
Lutte Anit-TB.

However, it should be noted that to cover hospitalisation costs at MF 200 per day, it would be necessary for there to be 6.3 million patient days per year—the equivalent of each person spending a day in hospital each year. Therefore, while people pay for hospital services the subsidy is very large. Also, it is most probably the case that 'transfer payments' are involved in the drug transactions of the Pharmacie d'Approvisionnement. In regularising these drug sales by officially charging at cost, MSP could save MF 1050 million per year or 30 per cent of its National Budget allocation. With this it is most probably the case that together with other charges and economies the health budget could double its coverage. In view of the relatively high social externalities associated with preventive medicine a crude but illustrative policy might be to charge for curative medicine while leaving preventive medicine free. If this were done the effective budget could be extended by 76 per cent since (see Table 4.13) 76 per cent of the National Budget is made over to curative measures. As an interim but practical measure the authorities should investigate a policy of charging 50 per cent of this total, i.e., 38 per cent of the MSP National Budget over a five year period. This would free resources for preventive health.

(v) Fiscal decentralisation:

We have already noted the considerable resource mobilisation that is generated at the local level through various self-help schemes and how cercle tax revenues have gradually been centralised. Appendix 4 draws attention to the fact that with the exception of the fourth region, the regional distribution of income in Mali is fairly uniform in the rural areas although this of course does not rule out the possibility of inter-regional disparities. Therefore, by and large, the regions' capacity to raise resources either to pay for health charges or for local fiscal purposes should be similar. The fact that so far the rural self-financing maternity model has only operated in the Sikasso region does not seem to be associated with that region's economic status. One would have to look for other explanations such as the ethnic structure of the region and its administrative and professional personnel.

Major policy questions are how far the Sikasso model is replicable, how can local resource mobilisation be encouraged, what is the appropriate role of government in this context? All of these questions raise the issue of fiscal and administrative decentralisation, and it must be asked whether resources would not be better mobilised and administered by reversing the trends towards centralisation.

The government itself is aware of this problem and based on studies of the National Commission for Administrative Reform the Military Committee for National Liberation issued an Ordinance (No. 77-44) on

12 July, 1977, which sought to clarify and reinforce the role of local administration, especially at the cercle level. In this context it is worth considering whether greater fiscal autonomy could be restored to the Regional Budget and whether the displaced taxe de cercle could be reinstated. Inevitably, such changes would be at the expense of the central fiscal authorities in Bamako and the issue is obviously highly political. Yet in issuing Ordinance 77-44, the government has launched a nation-wide debate to which the present sentiments naturally belong.

It was previously remarked that since the Direction Regionale de la Sante submits its budget directly to the Ministry of Finance via the Gouvernerat, MSP is unaware of these proposals and this can give rise to budgetary imbalances. There is an obvious need for co-ordination here and one possible solution would be to place the responsibility for investment and maintenance under one authority. Where the institution is regional the authority should be vested in the Regional Budget; where it is national it should be vested in the National Budget. For example regional hospitals, AM, PMI, etc. would most probably be better administered entirely at the regional level. This clearly is not the occasion to review how fiscal authonomy at the regional level might be achieved— at the very least the regions should not be required to pool their resources either directly or indirectly as they do at present. However, the taxe de cercle if reinstated would provide a source of revenue at the cercle level to finance a variety of health and other public services. Indeed, evidence suggests that there is a considerable fiscal consensus at the cercle level, that it is at this level that people perceive that they will receive benefits from their taxes. Already, the Sikasso rural health model indicates that the will and even some of the institutions are there, and there are indications of similar developments in other regions, especially the second and fifth.

The government is considering the establishment of a Health Fund along the line of its other special funds such as the Road Fund. This issue was raised in the five year plan and is currently under review. This development may be interpreted as an effort to decentralise the State Budget. However, in principle and with proper budgetary management a separate Health Fund should not be necessary. Such independent funds run the risk of allocating resources into areas long after it has ceased to be appropriate. The authorities would do far better to seek forms of decentralisation along the lines that have been indicated.

Notes

1   The information contained in this chapter was current as of mid-1978.

2   Protection Maternelle et Infantile—a service of child welfare clinics.
3   Agence Médicale—general health centres.
4   Department of Sanitation, water supply, etc.
5   A nationwide service to combat certain endemic diseases.
6   The official supply organisation for drugs.
7   In 1977 a seventh region of Tombouctou has been created out of the region of Gao.
8   The Pharmacie Populaire is a parastatal which is primarily run along commercial lines.
9   Keita assumed power when Mali became independent in 1960 but was deposed in 1967. The present military regime has been in control since then.
10   Village health educators and administers of first aid.
11   Population 90,253.
12   Population 46,088.
13   The norm is established by regressing per capita health expenditures (X) on income per capita (Y) for 19 of the countries represented on Table 4.11. This produces:

$$X = 0.00424Y + 0.064$$
$$R = 0.36$$

For Mali the expected value of X = $1.09 (i.e. when Y is 100). The actual value of X = $1.70.

APPENDIX 1

List of projects in the five year plan 1974-1978

Health

Curative:

1 Renovation and extension of health centre at Mopti

   estimated cost MF 563.7 millions;
   to be financed by FED;
   completed;

2 Renovation of Point 'G' Hospital

   estimated cost MF 625 millions;
   to be financed by FAC;
   virtually completed;

3 Completion of hospital at Nioro

   estimated cost MF 312.5 millions, revised to MF 1410 millions;
   to be financed by FED;
   FED funds have been committed;

4 Health centre at Sikasso

   estimated cost MF 625 millions revised to MF 1000 millions in
      1976;
   to be financed by Denmark;
   no action since Danes only wanted to finance 25 per cent of costs;

5 Health centre at Kayes

   estimated cost at MF 312.5 millions revised to MF 1000 millions;
   as with Sikasso health centre;

6 Upgrading health centres at San and Tominian

   estimated cost for medico-surgery block and equipment MF 135
      millions;
   to be slipped until the next plan;

7 Modernisation of hospital at Kati

   estimated cost MF 312 millions;
   finance requested from a German religious group;
   request refused;

8   Upgrading of health centre at Koulikoro

estimated cost MF 275 millions;
finance requested from West Germany;
request refused;

9   Upgrading of health centre at Kita

estimated cost MF 600 millions;
finance requested from German religious groups;
request refused;

10 New hospital for Bamako

estimated cost MF 1250 millions;
French construction firm has offered a loan;
the government is considering the loan offer;

11 Creation of a Polyclinic in Bamako

estimated cost MF 625 millions;
finance requested from Denmark in 1976;
Danes will reconsider in 1978;

12 Creation of dispensaries and maternities on the outskirts of
    Bamako

estimated cost MF 662.5 millions revised in 1976 to MF 1000
    millions;
finance requested from FED;
FED has committed the funds;

13 Strengthening two health centres per year

at an estimated cost of MF 62.5 millions per centre of which
    60 per cent would be external finance;
UNICEF and Swiss are involved but very little has been done;

14 Repairs to sanitary buildings

to be financed out of the State budget at MF 62.5 millions per
    year;
funds committed;

15 Building and equipment for Insitutute of Traditional Medicine

estimated cost MF 100 millions;
funds committed by Saudi Arabia;
only MF 7 millions disbursed;

16   Laboratory equipment for hospitals

     estimated cost MF 65 millions;
     Saudi Arabia will disburse the funds in 1978;

17   Completion of laboratory for heavy solutions

     estimated cost MF 8.7 millions;
     completed;

18   Improvement of dental centres in Bamako

     estimated cost MF 62.5 millions;
     Saudi Arabia has committed funds for disbursement in 1978-9.

Preventive:

19   Equipment for Service des Maladies Transmissibles

     estimated cost MF 51.2 millions;
     financed by FAC;

20   Vaccination programme for La Lutte Anti-Tuberculeuse

     estimated cost MF 71.2 millions;
     UNICEF has provided MF 26.4 millions;

21   Buildings and equipment for public hygiene

     estimated cost MF 17.5 millions;
     some internal funds have been obtained;

22   Construction of PMI

     estimated cost of MF 62.5 per year;
     negotiations have taken place with VNFPA but have not been
     satisfactorily resolved;

23   Extension of medical school to the regions

     estimated cost MF 31.1 millions;
     no finance obtained;

24   Mental health services

     estimated cost MF 62.5 millions;
     no finance obtained;

25   First Aid Posts

     estimated cost MF 60 millions;
     Red Cross has provided some of these funds;

26   Equipment for sanitary education

estimated cost MF 156 millions;
MF 10.8 millions received from UNICEF and MF 12 millions
received from the Frederich Ebert Foundation;

27   Onchocerciasis programmes

financed by international agencies;

28   Study centre for integrated rural development

estimated cost MF 562.0 millions;
UNICEF has financed MF 196.4 millions and will most
probably finance the remainder;

29   PMI centres in Sikasso

estimated cost MF 200.5 millions;
financed by IDA for MF 136 millions;

30   PMI–community development centres in Haute-Vallée

estimated cost MF 60.0 millions;
part financed by IDA, the remainder by USAID.

Source: *Actualisation et Situation des Projects d'Investissement de la
Santé Publique au 31 Decembre 1978,* March 1977; Ministère
du Plan.

APPENDIX 2

The balance between curative and preventive health

Health projects may be disaggregated into those which are curative (C) and those which are preventive (P). To some extent these projects will be complements for each other since preventive schemes may be supportive of curative schemes and vise versa; to some extent they may be substitutes for each other since health status may be stabilised by substituting preventive for curative measures.

Public health policy should be to combine preventive and curative health measures in such a way that for a given budget, public health status is maximised. This policy problem and its solution are illustrated in the figure below.

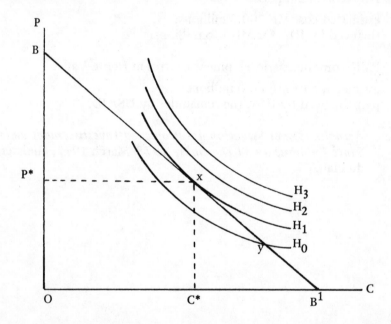

Optimal balance between preventive and curative health measures

The relationship between preventive and curative health measures may be expressed in a series of iso-health schedules H_0-H_3 where at various combinations of preventive and curative measures health status is constant. If the authorities are faced with a budget constraint such as BB^1 the optimal resource allocation between C and P will be C* and P* since at x health status is at a maximum.

It is probably the case that health expenditure in the developing countries is excessively weighted in favour of curative health and that consequently public health status is lower than it might otherwise be. For example, on the diagram the allocation at y represents a greater emphasis on curative health than the allocation at x and it implies that health status (H_0) is lower than at x (H_1). Indeed, as the emphasis on curative health increases public health status continues to deteriorate. The objective of health policy should be to determine the balance between curative and preventive measures which maximise health status.

On the diagram the iso-health schedules fan out as P increases for given C. This represents the assumption that there may be substantial favourable externalities with regard to preventive measures. Whereas curative medicine is on the whole concerned with the individual, preventive medicine tends to be concerned with society at large. As, for example, standards of hygiene improve, people will be less likely to contaminate and infect each other; the whole is more than the sum of its parts. By contrast curative medicine only tends to benefit the patients directly concerned. Especially in countries where standards of public health are low it is probable that the marginal returns to preventive health measures will be relatively high. As indicated on the diagram, such an assumption implies a high allocation of resources in favour of preventive health schemes.

APPENDIX 3

Optimal tax policies for drugs

Two kinds of drugs may be distinguished; essential drugs (E) and inessential drugs (N). The tax rate on the former is T_e and on the latter is T_n. Therefore, the tax take from drug sales will be:

$$T = ET_e + NT_n \qquad (1)$$

The respective demand curves for the two kinds of drugs may be written as:

$$E = A(P_e(1 + T_e))^{-a} \qquad (2)$$

$$N = B(P_n(1 + T_n))^{-b} \qquad (3)$$

Where P_e and P_n represent the basic drug prices and a and b are the (constant) price elasticities of demand.

While health ministers may wish to maximise E, finance ministers may stipulate that such policies be constrained by revenue objectives for $T = T^*$. Therefore, an issue in public health policy may be to maximise the consumption of essential drugs subject to such financial constraints, by picking the optimal combination of tax rates on the two kinds of drugs. Ideally, health ministers may wish to abolish tax rates on essential drugs ($T_e = 0$) or even subsidise them $T_e < 0$) but this might violate revenue objectives and taxes on inessential drugs might not be sufficiently large due to the pattern of demand elasticities.

Formally, the problem may be written as:

$$\text{Max } L = E + \lambda \, [ET_e + NT_n - T^*] \qquad (4)$$

$$(\text{w.r.t. } T_e, T_n)$$

Substituting equations (2) and (3) into (4), the first order conditions become:

$$\frac{\partial L}{\partial T_e} = -a\,AP_e^{-a}(1 + T_e)^{-(a+1)} + \lambda\,AP_e^{-a}[(1 + T_e)^{-a} - a\,T_e(1 + T_e)^{-(a+1)}] = 0 \quad (i)$$

$$\frac{\partial L}{\partial T_n} = BP_n^{-b}[(1 + T_n)^{-b} - b\,T_n(1 + T_n)^{-(b+1)}] = 0 \qquad (ii)$$

$$\frac{\partial L}{\partial \lambda} = T_e A(P_e(1 + T_e))^{-a} + T_n B(P_n(1 + T_n))^{-b} - T^* = 0 \qquad (iii)$$

*If $b < 1$ it will pay to set $T_n = -0$.

The solutions from equations (5) yield the optimal tax rates T_e^* and T_n^*. Notice that the model is recursive rather than simultaneous since the solution for T_n^* in equation (ii) does not depend on λ or T_e since from equation (i)

$$\lambda = \frac{a}{1 + T_e(1-a)} \qquad (6)$$

λ would be zero if $a = 0$, but if there is a zero elasticity of demand for essential drugs there is no problem in the first place. We, therefore, take the case where $a > 0$. For equation (ii) to hold it follows that:

$$T_n^* = 1/(b-1) \qquad (7)$$

This implies that the optimal tax rate on inessential drugs is entirely independent of the revenue objective and the elasticity of demand for essential drugs.* It also implies that the authorities should squeeze as much tax revenue as the market will bear from inessential drugs and then proceed to set the tax rate on essential drugs in such a way that the net revenue differential is made up. If at T_n^*, $NT_n^* > T^*$ it will be possible to subsidise essential drugs, i.e., $T_e^* < 0$. If $NT_n^* < T^*$ it will be necessary to tax essential drugs too.

Substituting from equation (7) implies that the revenue differential (R) is:

$$R = T^* - BP_n^{-b} b^{-b} (b-1)^{(b-1)} \qquad (8)$$

and the optimal tax rate on essential drugs may be solved from

$$T_e^* A(P_e(1 + T_e^*))^{-a} = R \qquad (9)$$

The condition for zero taxation on essential drugs is that $R = 0$ from equation (8).

*If $b < 1$ it will pay to set $T_n = \infty$

APPENDIX 4

The distribution of income in the rural areas of Mali

It is important for health planning purposes to determine the geographical distribution of health and income since richer areas may be able to afford to pay for certain medical services while poorer areas may well be in need of resource transfers to pay for health services. As a first approximation it seems sensible to focus on the regional distribution in Mali. However, such data do not exist and the Malians themselves have never attempted such an exercise. The latest available data are for GNP in 1973 but unfortunately the national accounts are not constructed from their regional components.

In this appendix an attempt is made to determine the regional distribution of income in the rural areas based on the limited data that are available. The objective is more the qualitative one of identifying the poorer and richer areas rather than the quantitative one of establishing reasonably precise magnitudes. One possible hypothesis might be that the per capita income distribution varies directly with the volume of rainfall since agricultural output obviously depends on the volume of rainfall. This would imply that the south was relatively rich. However, the focus should be on productivity rather than output and there is no prior reason why rainfall and productivity should be correlated if the distribution of the population also happens to reflect the distribution of rainfall. Indeed, the exercise below bears out this supposition.

The calculations reported are based on a survey of agricultural output in 1973 and a survey of livestock in 1975. Unfortunately the former survey will have been distorted by the drought and it is possible that the livestock figures in 1975 are still affected in the wake of the drought. It is therefore assumed that the distribution of agricultural output in 1975 was the same as in 1973 and it is on this basis that revenues are calculated. However, if the Sahelian regions suffered more on account of the drought this methodology would bias estimates of regional income distribution in favour of the non-Sahelian regions.

Off-take ratios are assumed for livestock based on West African practice and the income from livestock reflects the value of milk production from the animals. For want of a better assumption, agricultural production is valued according to an unweighted average of the official and unofficial prices. The coverage of rural production is extensive enough and it is unlikely that omitted items will significantly prejudice the calculations. The calculations omit fruit production in the south, but they also omit fish production in the north. In Mopti, for example, it is estimated that fish production averages at about 30 kg/capita and in 1975 the price of fresh fish was about MF 550/kg. On the other hand, since the population figures are based on the 1976 census and the census date was 16 December, it is possible that the population in the south was bloated by migrants from the north seeking the moister agricultural areas. This would tend to bias calculations of income distribution in favour of the north.

The table below ranks the per capita income distribution as follows:

Segou
Kayes
Mopti
Gao
Bamako
Sikasso

i.e., the Sahelian regions take second, third and fourth places. However, it should be pointed out that the figures for all the regions except Segou are not significantly different from each other. It is therefore more appropriate to conclude that in 1975 the regional distribution of income was fairly uniform across these five regions. Since 1975, the terms of trade have moved sharply in favour of the regions producing livestock which would imply that (ceteris paribus) the distribution of income will have moved in favour of the north. Similar qualitative results that the distribution of rural income is not biassed in favour of the areas of greater rainfall have been found for Chad supporting the hypothesis that the population distribution tends to arbitrage away productivity differentials.

It should of course be emphasised that certain inter-regional areas may be relatively deprived. For example in the fifth region in 1972 when average cattle per head was 1.6, the ratios in the cercles of Djenne and Bandiagara were 0.7 and 0.4 respectively reflecting the low ratios of Peuhl in those areas. However, for the country as a whole the regional distribution of rural per capita income seems uniform enough.

Estimates of regional distribution of income in rural Mali

Year		Kayes	Bamako	Sikasso	Segou	Mopti	Gao
1973	Output						
	Agriculture (tonnes)[a]						
	Millet, sorghum and maize	123501	121264	99471	132688	136186	8569
	Rice	27	8938	7813	89055	21904	2973
	Cotton	–	4298	21753	3243	–	–
	Groundnuts	76821	3357	13204	9590	4820	–
1975	Livestock[b] (head)						
	Cattle	50700	555000	630000	433000	1170000	620000
	Small stock	779000	668000	445000	779000	2449000	6010000
	Value (MF millions)						
	Agriculture						
	Millet, sorghum and maize[1] (MF 36/kg)	8388.7	8236.7	6756.6	9012.8	8910.7	582.1
	Rice[2] (MF 47/kg)	4.3	1400.0	1224.0	13952.0	3431.7	465.7
	Cotton[3] (MF 90/kg)	–	768.8	3893.1	580.2	–	–
	Groundnuts[4] (MF 60/kg)	6983.8	305.2	1200.4	871.8	438.2	–
	Livestock						
	Cattle (MF 5440/head)	275.8	3019.2	3427.2	2355.5	6364.8	3372.8
	Small stock (MF 1200/head)	934.8	801.6	534.0	934.8	2938.8	7212.0
	Total	16587.4	14531.5	17035.3	27707.1	22084.2	11632.6
	Rural population (1976)	827135	891157	112483	919723	1180298	693059
	Average rural revenue per capita	20054	16306	15145	30125	18711	16784

Price assumptions:
Agricultural output: average of free and controlled prices in 1975.
Cattle: 10 per cent off-take rate at MF 40000/head + 24 per cent milking rate at MF 50/litre and 120 litres/cow.
Small stock: 30 per cent off-take rate at MF 3000/head + 30 per cent milking rate at MF 50/litre and 20 litres/head.

1 1973 output scaled in line with 88.7 per cent increase in production in 1975.
2 1973 output scaled in line with 23.3 per cent increase in production in 1975.
3 1973 output scaled in line with 98.7 per cent increase in production in 1975.
4 1973 output scaled in line with 51.5 per cent increase in production in 1975.

Sources: a Rapport de l'Enquête Agricole 1973-4, page 22; Direction Nationale du Plan et de la Statistique.
b Statistiques du Bétail et de la Viande 1976, page 2; Office Malien du Bétail et de la Viande.

92

5 The cost of nutrition in Indonesia and the poverty line

Introduction

The main objective in this chapter is to calculate the cost of diet adequacy in Indonesia using the technique of linear programming. A number of nutritional targets are set and the prices and nutritional content for a range of Indonesian staples are obtained. The linear programme computes the minimum cost combination of these staples that satisfies all of the nutritional objectives.

This optimal diet is of course a theoretical minimum which in practice would be difficult to achieve for a number of reasons. First, the simple methodology followed does not take account of the numerous traditional recipes and dietary combinations practiced by the Indonesians. Secondly, man does not eat for nutrition alone and the minimum cost diet might not be sufficiently appetising. However, for the very poor where the incidence of malnutrition will tend to be greatest and where the luxury of appetising diets can be least afforded, the theoretical minimum assumes a more immediate relevance. Nevertheless, even as a first approximation of the cost of nutritional adequacy in Indonesia the exercise seems worthwhile in the face of numerous reports of malnutrition. Moreover, this first approximation is particularly interesting since the minimum cost diet is calculated to be fairly low. Another feature of the minimum cost diet is the relative cost inefficiency of the traditional staple, rice, which is counterbalanced by the cost efficiency of cassava and maize.

Since about 80 per cent of the expenditure of the poor goes on food items this approach may be used to derive a poverty line below which people will run the risk of malnutrition and related symptoms of poverty. In the past 'poverty' has been defined in quite arbitrary terms[1] and without any formal relationship with the symptoms of poverty. Another approach has been to take the food consumption basket of the poor from the 1969/70 *Socio-Economic Survey* and to scale up the volume of consumption to produce a satisfactory number of calories. On this basis a 'poverty line' of $90 per capita was calculated at 1976 prices. The obvious advantage of this methodology over the linear programming approach would be that it took into account the tastes of the poor. However, it has been argued[2] that the *Socio-Economic Survey* seriously understates the consumption of cassava and sweet potato in particular in which case the methodology is as unreliable as the survey upon which it is based. The linear programming approach suggests a poverty line for Indonesia in the region of $60 per capita (at mid-1976 prices). This contrasts with Ahluwalia's figure of about $104.

Before calculating the cost of nutritional adequacy a brief description of the state of nutrition in Indonesia is presented.

The extent of malnutrition

Aggregative nutrition surveys in Indonesia do not indicate a national malnutrition problem. For example in 1964 estimates for middle income families (per capita expenditure of Rp 50,000 per year at 1976 prices) in Java and Madura indicate daily per capita calorie intake of 2,113 calories per day and an intake of 26 grams of protein.[3] Higher expenditure groups consumed slightly more protein (31.8 grams per day) but on the whole tended to spend their money on more expensive foods such as eggs, fish and beef. In the light of the nutritional objectives described below, these figures do not indicate an aggregative malnutrition problem at least as far as calories and proteins are concerned.

Similarly, Edmunson's study[4] of three Javanese villages in 1969 does not indicate any aggregative signs of malnutrition with the possible exception of vitamin A where average per capita consumption was 81 per cent of the target discussed below. However, even here, given the uncertainty about the appropriate target this figure most probably does not constitute a statistically significant deficiency.

At the disaggregated level, however, it would seem that Indonesia has a serious malnutrition problem especially in relation to the very young and the old. Edmunson found[5] that children after weaning and until the age of six suffered extensively from protein-calorie malnutrition as well as deficiency in riboflavin, and that people over the age of forty-five seemed poorly nourished. In 1974 a WHO sponsored team reported that protein-calorie malnutrition among Indonesian children below the age of two was particularly severe and pregnant and lactating women were another vulnerable group. These factors combine to determine a large part of the high infant mortality rate of 110-150 per thousand.[6]

The incidence of vitamin A deficiency in Indonesia is among the highest in the world especially among children and a recent study has shown that between 50 to 80 per cent of those children surveyed in North and West Sumatra, East Java and Bali were found to have goiter which is related to iodine deficiency.[7] Indonesia also has the highest country incidence of nutritional anaemia ever recorded in a male population during nonfamine conditions. Among a sample taken in 1973 and 1974[8] the incidence among male workers was 28-52 per cent. The incidence among nonpregnant women was 35-85 per cent and among pregnant women it was 50-92 per cent.

The extent of malnutrition is selective in two aspects rather than a general problem. First, children emerge as the most vulnerable group. Secondly, vitamin A and iron are not adequately consumed. Nevertheless it must seriously be considered how far Indonesia's economic backwardness is related to the stunted intellectual and physical development of her children who are inadequately fed and who eventually grow up into the working population.

Nutrient targets

In the present study eight nutrients are explicitly entered into the analysis.[9] These are: calories, protein, vitamin A, iron, thiamin, riboflavin, vitamin C and niacin. Additional nutrients such as iodine, vitamin B-12, the trace elements etc. are excluded from the analysis given the limitations (discussed below) of our choice of staples. In tropical climates vitamin D is provided naturally by the sun. These nutrients provide a sufficiently rich range in their own right and go well beyond the more traditional evaluations that concentrate on calories and protein.

Unfortunately no unambiguous targets for nutrients may be provided since there is uncertainty about what requirements should be. Furthermore, nutrients are interactive and should not be considered as independent targets. For example absorption of vitamin A is enhanced by consumption of vitamin E, and metabolic rates may also be affected by the chemical reaction of different nutrients. It is also recognised that individual needs of different nutrients will vary from person to person in which case the figures suggested are intended to be broad averages which are likely to fulfill bodily needs of the average individual.

Given their smaller stature and the hot climate in Indonesia, Indonesians are likely to require less calories and protein than their counterparts in the cooler climates of the westernised countries. However, their requirements for the remaining nutrients would tend to be broadly the same. The daily requirements[10] set out in Table 5.1 are for a family of five based on a mother and father, one adolescent, a 7-10 year old and a 4-6 year old. The mother is assumed to be lactating or pregnant for 40 per cent of the time and the weights between boys and girls (since they have different nutritional requirements) are equal.

95

Table 5.1

Daily nutritional requirements per capita

	Calorie	Protein	Vitamin A	Iron	Thiamin	Riboflavin	Vitamin C	Niacin
		grams net	IU	m.grams	m.grams	m.grams	m.grams	m.grams
1950		30	4000	12	1.14	1.4	4.0	15.4

The protein requirement is expressed in net terms i.e., it is the protein to be absorbed by the body since in most cases the protein content of food is not fully absorbed. The status of these targets requires careful interpretation. Failure to achieve any or all of them does not necessarily imply that the individual will suffer. Rather, he will increase his chances of malnutrition. In other words the targets on average will guarantee an adequate degree of safety from malnutrition.

Nutritional content of food

Table 5.2 sets out the nutritional content of eighteen different Indonesian staples and their prices. The prices are based on the 'prices of 12 food articles in the rural markets of Java and Madura' and 'average retail prices of goods in rural markets by provinces of Java and Madura' as published in the various issues of the *Indikator Ekonomi*. Where appropriate the different provincial prices have been averaged in which case the minimum cost diet would strictly relate to rural market areas in Java and Madura. The analysis and prices are expressed in terms of mid-1976 rupiah.

The nutritional coefficients have been taken from the Food Consumption Table for Use in Southeast Asia as published by the FAO and the US Department of Health, Education and Welfare in December 1972. For example one kilogram of rice contains 1,460 calories, 14.7 grams of protein net, no vitamin A, two miligrams of iron and so on. Since only about 67 per cent of the protein of rice is absorbed by the body, the gross protein content is 22 grams. Since in Indonesia rice is invariably cooked the nutritional coefficients have been calculated for cooked rice. It is interesting to note that in the case of uncooked rice there are 3,570 calories and 47.6 grams of protein, i.e., cooking destroys much of the nutritional value of rice. A brief commentary on the nature of these staples is provided in Table 5.2.

Tempe is a traditional Indonesian dish[11] based almost totally on soyabeans and for present purposes the price has been based on the price of soyabeans. The price of saridele which is another traditional dish based on peanuts and soyabeans is an average of the prices of peanuts and soyabeans.

96

Table 5.2

Nutritional properties and cost of staples
(units per kilogram)

	Price Rupiah/kg	Calories	Protein grams	Vitamin A IU	Iron mg	Thiamin mg	Riboflavin mg	Vitamin C mg	Niacin mg	Food description
Rice	140	3,570 a	14.7 b	0	2	0.4	0.1	0	10	Cooked
Maize	75	3,550	44.6	2,250	28	2.9	1.1	0	21	Mixed white and yellow, ground.
Peanuts	295	3,030	97.5	330	21	9.7	1.8	110	97	Shelled and raw.
Soyabeans	173	1,490	135	500	100	170	0	0	0	'Tempe': mold treated pressed soyabean cake.
Saridele	234	4,460	210	20,000 c	40	7	100	100	0	Mixture of soyabeans and peanuts.
Dry cassava	27	3,330 d	10	0	10	0.6	0.5	0	8	Edible portion.
Fresh cassava	17	1,350 d	7.5	0	9	0.5	0.4	340	6	Raw yellow edible portion. (NB: boiling eliminates Vitamin A)
Sweet potato	30	1,150	7	28,000 e	9	1.2	0.5	300	6	Unclassified, salted and dried.
Fish	315	1,930	360	0	9	0.8	3.1	0	46	As purchased, cooked whole.
Hen's eggs	600	1,450	115	17,330	28	0.9	3.3	0	1	As purchased, cooked whole.
Duck's eggs	800	1,860	127	11,080	29	1.6	3.3	0	1	As purchased, raw.
Bananas	120	630	6	2,330	5	0.2	0.2	90	4	Edible portion, raw.
Buffalo	942 f	1,200	177	180	33	0.6	1,550	0	350	As purchased, medium fat, raw.
Beef	833	2,180	138	400	18	0.5	2.9	0	36	Crude, brown.
Sugar	145	3,890	9	0	58	0.5	1	0	3	Green, fresh.
Beans	70	270	13	5,116	11	0.5	1	170	6	As purchased.
Chili	266	1,000	30	95,000	31	3.2	4.5	840	22	As purchased.
Spinach	38	140	13	44,916	30	0.5	1.7	420	5	

a Cooking may affect the vitamin coefficients.
b 47.6 raw.
c Vitamin enriched.
d 3,490 as chips, but other nutrients are lost.
e Boiling eliminates Vitamin A.
f Assumes 20 per cent refuse rate.

With the exception of saridele these primary foods will be combined in almost inumerable combinations through which their final nutritional properties might be modified in some cases, especially when heated to high temperatures. A further limitation is that a large number of foods are not on the list due to lack of price data. Nevertheless, the list as it stands is sufficiently comprehensive in relation to the number of nutrient objectives which have been set.

Optimisation procedure

The objective of the exercise is to find the combination of these eighteen staples which minimise the cost of satisfying the nutrient requirements set out in Table 5.1. This optimal combination will determine the minimum cost diet. The cost of the diet (C) may be written as the sum of the products of the unit prices of the different foods (Pi) and the number of units (Qi) of each food:

$$C = \sum_{i=1}^{18} Pi\ Qi$$

This cost is to be minimised subject to two sets of constraints. The first set of constraints requires that the quantities of food cannot be negative, i.e.:

$$Qi \geq 0 \qquad i = 1, 2, ..., 18$$

The second set of constraints requires that the nutrient targets (Tj) be at least attained, i.e.:

$$\sum_{i=1}^{18} aij\ Qi \geq Tj \qquad j = 1, 2, ..., 8$$

This is a conventional linear programming problem for which solutions are provided.

Results

In the base run (when all eighteen foods are considered and no additional constraints are set) only four of the eighteen foods were involved in the optimal or least cost diet. Table 5.3 sets out the nature of this diet.

Table 5.3

Least cost diet: base run

	Weight kg	Calorie	Protein grams	Vitamin A IU	Iron mg	Thiamin mg	Riboflavin mg	Vitamin C mg	Niacin mg	Cost Rp
Fresh cassava	2.14856	2900.5	16.11	0	19.34	1.074	0.86	730	12.89	36.5
Fish	.04361	84.2	15.7	0	0.39	.03	0.14	0	2	13.7
Buffalo	.00016	0.2	0	0	0	0	0.24	0	0.6	0.15
Spinach	.08905	12.5	1.16	4000	2.67	.04	0.15	37.4	0.44	3.38
Total	2.28138	2997.4	33	4000	22.41	1.154	1.4	767.9	15.4	53.73

Note: Discrepancies due to rounding.

Since the nutrient requirements are regarded as minima the diet is permitted to include more of the various nutrients than is minimally required. The diet reported on Table 5.3 has a 54 per cent excess of calories, an 87 per cent excess of iron, a 1.2 per cent excess of thiamin and an eighteen-fold excess of Vitamin C. These surpluses will not be harmful to health.[12] From an economic viewpoint these surpluses are not strictly inefficient since it pays to overshoot certain nutrient targets to arrive at minimum cost combinations with respect to other targets. In principle the addition of extra food items would raise the degrees of freedom in the minimum cost set and the minimum cost diet would involve lower percentage surpluses.

The outstanding feature of Table 5.3 is the dependence on fresh cassava which provides all the essential calories, iron, Vitamin C, half the protein, about all the thiamin, 84 per cent of the niacin and 60 per cent of the riboflavin requirements. Spinach provides all the requirements of Vitamin A and fish the balance of the protein requirement. The cost of this diet is a bit less than Rp 54 per day per head.

This and the other dietary combinations that are discussed are intended to be indicative of the basis of the diet strategy that will be adequate and cheap rather than a prescription for detailed diet adequacy where all of the manifold nutrients are taken into consideration, e.g., the trace elements, iodine and other vitamin and mineral complexes. Some of these requirements will be satisfied even in the indicative diet. Others will have to be supplemented at a small price through the consumption of small quantities of other foods in which these nutrients are present. Nevertheless, the eight nutrients under review (and especially the first four) are singled out for analysis because of their relative prominence as nutritional objectives.

Indicative as this diet may be, an obvious shortcoming is the volume of cassava consumption of over 2 kg per day. Later on additional dietary constraints are composed in the form of a ceiling on the weight[13] of food that can be eaten comfortably. Nevertheless, Table 5.3 indicates the economic efficiency of fresh cassava as a source of all the nutrients under review with the exception of Vitamin A. This result requires qualification since cassava is sometimes regarded as the 'bete noire' of staples in deference to rice. From a volumetric point of view cassava is an inefficient food, but given that the price of fresh cassava by weight is an eighth of the price of rice its efficiency from an economic standpoint is considerable.

The relative economic inefficiencies of the staples excluded from the solution of the minimum cost diet may be measured by taking the percentage price fall required to enter them into the optimum solution set. These percentage price falls are set out in Table 5.4.

Table 5.4

Economic inefficiency of foods: base run

Rice	79	Dry cassava	16	Beef	81
Maize	5	Sweet potato	4	Sugar	92
Peanuts	13	Hen's eggs	86	Beans	68
Soyabeans	52	Duck's eggs	89	Chili	60
Saridele	41	Banana	89		

For example the price of rice must fall by 79 per cent before rice enters the solution for the minimum cost diet. In other words the nutritional roles of rice are being much more economically fulfilled by the competing staples. In the context of the base run rice emerges as a luxury food as do eggs, bananas, beef, sugar, beans, chili and soyabeans in the sense that their respective nutritional roles are provided considerably more cheaply by competing staples. Maize and sweet potato lie just outside the solution set and dry cassava and peanuts a little way further. Given the confidence limits about the price assumptions, these four foods would probably tend to feature in a cost-efficient diet for practical purposes.

The diet in the base run involved the consumption of more than 2 kg of food per day by the average household member. At the very best this will constitute an uncomfortable if not impossible task. However, it should be realised that the Indonesian practice of mixing staples which has the effect in some cases of increasing their nutritional efficiency will reduce this constraint.[14] Unfortunately there is no consensus as to what constitutes a comfortable diet volume especially in the context of Southeast Asia. Edmunson's observations[15] imply that the weight of food consumed is in the order of 1 kg per day. In the next exercise therefore the minimum cost diet is constrained by a weight limitation of 1.4 kg of food per day.[16] Table 5.5 sets out the least cost diet in this case.

The most important feature of the table is that the cost of the weight-constrained diet is only slightly more than one rupiah greater than the cost in the base run. This is attributed to the fairly close substitutability between maize and fresh cassava, both from the point of view of price and nutritional properties. The minimum cost diet in this case requires 0.41442 kg of maize and smaller quantities of everything else with the exception of buffalo meat which, in any case, is only required in very small quantities as a source of riboflavin. Less spinach is required because maize is also a source of Vitamin A. The percentage excess of calories, iron and Vitamin C are lower, but there is now a greater excess of thiamin than previously was the case.

Table 5.5

Least cost diet: weight constrained run

	Weight kg	Calorie	Protein grams	Vitamin A IU	Iron mg	Thiamin mg	Riboflavin mg	Vitamin C mg	Niacin mg	Cost Rp
Maize	.41442	1471.2	18.48	932.4	11.6	1.2	0.86	0	3.6	31.1
Fresh cassava	.89806	1203.4	6.73	0	8.1	0.45	0.36	305.4	5.4	15.3
Fish	.01902	36.7	6.85	0	0.2	0.01	0.06	0	0.9	6.0
Buffalo	.00026	0.3	0.05	.5	0	0	0.4	0	0.1	0.2
Spinach	.06829	9.6	0.89	3067.3	2.0	.03	.11	28.7	0.3	2.6
Total	1.4	2730.1	33	4000	21.9	1.7	1.4	334	15.4	55

Notes: Descrepancies due to rounding.

Table 5.6

Economic inefficiency of foods: weight constrained run

Rice	78	Dry cassava	13	Banana	89
Peanuts	3	Sweet potato	2	Beef	80
Soyabeans	56	Hen's eggs	87	Sugar	93
Saridele	45	Duck's eggs	90	Beans	68
				Chili	58

The basic feature of Table 5.6 is that rice continues to be economically inefficient and that peanuts and sweet potato are on the verge of entering the minimum cost solution set. Changes in the values on Table 5.6 from their values in Table 5.4 reflect the nutritional weight efficiency of various foods.

Conclusions

The calculations indicate that diet adequacy can be achieved for about Rp 55 per day at mid-1976 prices. Indeed, this diet would exceed nutrient requirements in certain cases. According to the Socio-Economic Survey conducted in 1969/70, 25 per cent of those surveyed in Indonesia spent less than Rp 55 per day on food.[17] By the end of 1976, real GNP per capita is likely to have grown by about 40 per cent. If the distribution of income and expenditure is broadly as it was in 1969/70[18] and relative food prices were unchanged, probably about 10 per cent of the population would presently be spending less than Rp 55 per day on food.[19] Several more years of economic growth would tend to reduce this figure even further.

If it is assumed that 80 per cent of per capita expenditure is allocated to food, the linear programming approach to the determination of the 'poverty line' suggests a figure of about $60 per capita. Another aspect of the analysis is that rice is an expensive staple and that maize and cassava are relatively cheap and effective as the basis for the poor man's diet.

Notes

1   See e.g. M. S. Ahluwalia 'Income Inequality: Some Dimensions of the Problem' in *Redistribution with Growth*, H. Chenery, et al, Oxford University Press, 1975, pp.10-11.
2   See D. Dapice 'Income Distribution in Indonesia', SEADAG, May 1976.

3   Data based on *Survey Sosial Ekonomi Nasional,* 1969/70, *Biro Pusat Statistik, Jakarta, 1973,* and Food Consumption Tables for Use in East Asia, FAO/WHO.

4   W. C. Edmunson, *Land Food and Work in East Java,* New England Monographs in Geography No. 4, March 1976, page 73. Edmunson's nutrient targets differ in several respects from those discussed below which are based on more recent data.

5   Ibid., pp. 75-76.

6   If survivors of protein-calorie malnutrition are not treated before the age of two there is a high risk for permanent impairment to physical and mental development. Many of the happy and healthy six year olds that the unassuming visitor to Indonesia sees are in fact eight or nine year olds! See C. S. Rose and P. Gyorgy 'Malnutrition in Children in Indonesia, *Resources on the Technological Development,* H. W. Beers (editor), Lexington, The University Press of Kentucky, 1970.

7   See D. A. Nain et al, 'The Problems of Epidemic Goiter in Some Parts of Sumatera, Java, Bali, Indonesia', *Second Asian Nutrition Congress,* Manila 1973. See also A. Querido, 'A Proposal for the Eradication of Goiter and Cretinism in Indonesia', University of Leiden, 1973. Querido shows that 10 million people are affected by goiter, 100,000 by cretinism and another 500,000 are in the early stages of cretinism in Indonesia.

8   See D. Karyadi on S. S. Basta, 'Nutrition and Health of Indonesian Construction Workers', IBRD Staff Paper No. 152, 1973. Also S. S. Basta and A. Churchill, 'Iron Deficiency and the Productivity of Adult Males in Indonesia', IBRD Staff Paper No. 175, 1974. They show that the productivity of anaemic workers is at least 20 per cent lower than productivity of normal workers.

9   For a useful lay introduction to nutrition see J. D. Kirschmann, *'Nutrition Almanac',* McGraw Hill Book Company, 1975.

10   See the chart in Kirschmann, op.cit., pp. 237-238. See also *Energy and Protein Requirements,* FAO/WHO Rome, 1973.

11   See Edmunson, op.cit., pp.67-72 for a description of Indonesian dietary habits. Also see Mely G. Tan et al, 'Social and Cultural Aspects of Food Patterns and Food Habits in Five Rural Areas in Indonesia', LEKNAS, Jakarta, Mimeo, 1970.

12   Indeed some experts believe a much higher dosage of Vitamin C is desirable. See Kirschmann, op.cit., p.44.

13   A volume constraint would have been appropriate too but this was not practicable under the circumstances. However, a weight constraint would be a reasonable first order approximation to a true consumption constraint.

14   See Edmunson, op.cit., pp. 57-68.

15   See Edmunson, op.cit., p. 68.

16   In practice food mixing will reduce the effective constraint towards 1 kg.

17   Survey Sosial Ekonomi Nasional, Biro Pusat Statistik, Jakarta, 1973. Combining Table 1, p. 1, and Table 5.2A, p. 118. These calculations assume that mid-1976 prices are 2.91 times early 1970 prices.

18   For further discussion, see H. W. Arndt, 'Development and Equality: the Indonesian Case', *World Development,* February/March 1975, pp. 77-90.

19   Applying the tables referred to in the *Survey Sosial Ekonomi Nasional.*

PART II

STUDIES IN MIGRATION

6 Land settlement principles and the economics of transmigration

The economics of transmigration

The economics of transmigration are essentially concerned with two main questions:

(a) What, if any, are the likely contributions of transmigration to Indonesia's economic development?

(b) If transmigration has a positive role to play in Indonesia, what are the economic principles upon which the design of transmigration policy should be based?

The section headed 'The Indonesian economy and the other islands' discusses the economic aspects of the previous interest and concern with transmigration. In particular it is asked why in the context of the history of transmigration and the dubious economic and social contribution of transmigration in the past (even at a time when more productive lands for transmigration were available) is transmigration still considered to be of importance in the context of Indonesia's economic and social future.

The section headed 'The macroeconomic context of transmigration' discusses the first question and suggests that especially in the light of the various land reviews, agriculturally based transmigration promises to contribute little to Indonesia's economic development both in absolute terms and relative to alternative strategies of economic development in Indonesia. The section headed 'Land settlement, the role of government and the design of transmigration projects' addresses itself to the second question and suggests that government directed transmigration as a form of land settlement is a high risk strategy and that lower levels of government participation are likely to improve the economic prospects of transmigration. Instead the authorities should limit their participation to improving the access to capital where legitimate and to providing the infrastructure which will have the effect of narrowing the diversions between private and social settlement costs.

This would provide the basis for what might be called the 'minimal infrastructure' approach to transmigration—where the authorities after having favourably assessed the economic potential of an unsettled area install low cost access roads, bridges, etc. (i.e. infrastructure which so far has impeded successful settlement) and then await the unassisted settlement of the area.

At this point the authorities should provide the inputs over which they effectively happen to have control, e.g. fertilizers, pesticides, extension services, planting materials, etc. In addition, prospective settlers, even those that are in need of financial assistance, should bear an appropriate share of the risks involved in settlement.

At all times it is important to focus on the resource costs to Indonesia rather than the narrow financial costs of the various projects to the government. While inevitably the financial aspects impose a cash flow constraint on the government, the economic contribution must be judged by its efficiency in terms of resource utilisation. Therefore, the lower government involvement of the 'minimal infrastructure' approach does not in itself imply a lower project cost in terms of resource use. However, the economic analysis that follows would suggest this to be the case.

The Indonesian economy and the other islands

Economic indicators

Historically, transmigration has been regarded as a solution to the problems of overpopulation and low productivity in Java. The fear has always been that the pressure due to population growth on Javanese land resources in particular would imply declining productivity and per capita income trends. On the other hand, the other islands were relatively unpopulated and it was thought that transmigrating people from the 'overcrowded' parts of Java to the open spaces of the other islands would, along with birth control encouragement, be an important response to population pressures in Java.

Frequently, the proponents of transmigration refer to the apparent economic disparities between Java, Bali and Madura and the other islands, which transmigration would narrow in a socially desirable fashion. The most striking feature in these respects is most probably the geographical distribution of the population since, as shown in Table 6.1, Java has a population concentration which is about 12 times greater than the next most densely populated island.

Between 1930 and 1976 the Javanese population grew by about 105 per cent or at an annual average rate of 1.6 per cent. Rates of population growth in other parts of Indonesia are considerably higher than this at 2.2 per cent over the same period. In other words there has been a systematic tendency towards a greater degree of equality in the distribution of the population for which transmigration seems to have borne little responsibility.

Table 6.1

Population density

	Population (millions)			Density per sq.km.		
	1930	1971	1976 (est.)	1930	1971	1976
Java, Bali and Madura	42.8	78.7	87.7	311	571	637
Sumatra	8.3	21.0	24.3	18	44	51
Kalimantan	2.2	5.2	5.9	4	10	11
Sulawesi	4.2	8.6	9.8	22	45	51
Other	3.1	6.6	7.5	5	12	13
Total	60.6	120.1	135.2	32	63	71

Should the historic growth rate of the Javanese population continue, by 2000 it will have risen by 53 per cent or 40 million (from 1971) and the pressure on the land will have further increased. Thus despite the fact that Indonesian, (and particularly Javanese) population growth is among the slowest in the developing world it is feared that the pressure on Javanese land resources will become even greater than at present.

Table 6.2

Regional economic contributions

%	Java & Bali	Sumatra	Kalimantan	Sulawesi	Other
Population a	65.5	17.6	4.3	7.1	5.5
GDP (nonoil) a	60.6	22.3	7.9	5.3	3.9
Rice production b	60.6	21.5	4.9	7.3	5.7
Agriculture c	55.1	22.3	11.7	6.0	4.9
Construction c	65.3	18.6	3.3	4.3	8.5
Transport c	51.5	36.6	3.5	5.9	2.5
Manufacturing c	79.9	14.5	1.9	2.5	1.2

a From H. Esmara, 'Regional Income Disparities', *Bulletin of Indonesian Economic Studies,* March 1975, p. 45. Data for 1972.

b *Production of Food Crops in Indonesia,* Biro Pusat Statistik, Jakarta, September 1975, Table 1. Data for 1973.

c Constructed from Table 3, p.119 in *'The Economic Development of West Sumatera',* by H. Esmara, Research Department of Economics, Andalas University, Padang, August 1974.

Table 6.2 shows that Java and Bali, while having 65.5 per cent of the population 1972 accounted for slightly less than their proportionate share of GDP, implying that GDP per capita is on average significantly lower in Java and Bali than it is in Sumatra —by about 10 per cent. Sumatra and Kalimantan have a strong agricultural base; however, the agricultural sector has only been growing by about 4 per cent per year. The fast growing sectors are construction and transportation and

111

construction has a high employment elasticity. Java and Bali have a disproportionately large share of manufacturing, but this sector has had a growth rate equal to the overall growth rate of GDP.

Table 6.3 below shows the real regional growth rates over the period 1968-72. The figure for Kalimantan is swollen by the growth in the timber sector in East Kalimantan. Otherwise, the growth rate would have been about 4 per cent per year. Taking into account the lower rate of population growth in Java, the table suggests that real per capita income growth in Java has not been out of line with developments in the other islands. Thus, while real GDP per capita in Sumatra is about 8 per cent greater than in Java, the growth rate in per capita GDP in Java has been about 4.2 per cent, and in Sumatra about 4.4 per cent.

Table 6.3

Regional growth rates 1968-1972

	Java	Sumatra	Kalimantan	Sulawesi	Indonesia
Percentage per annum	5.8	6.6	10.8	3.0	6.3

Source: H. Esmara, *The Economic Development of West Sumatera* p. 136.

The roles of the various economic sectors, as shown in Table 6.4, suggest a further problem concerning the economic future of Indonesia. The agricultural sector which is by far the largest sector accounting for 43 per cent of GDP and 64 per cent of the labour force is also one of the slowest growing sectors. In addition a significant part of this growth may be attributed to the Green Revolution which has been associated with the breakdown of 'agricultural involution' in Java and its associated dishoarding of labour.[2] Therefore it is likely that the rate of growth in agricultural employment has been very low if not negative. Combining the growth rates shown in Table 6.3 and the associated employment— output elasticities[3] implies that the growth in agricultural employment has been about 0.8 per cent per year whereas the fastest growing sector has been construction where employment growth has been of the order of 13½ per cent per year, but where the share of the labour force is only 1.6 per cent. Since the labour force is projected to grow (between 1971 and 1981) at an annual rate of about 2½ per cent[4] Table 6.4 suggests a considerable shortfall in the demand of labour.

The objective of transmigration in this context would be that by opening up agricultural employment in the other islands some of this shortfall could be made up. Nevertheless, a sense of historical perspective is required since 'Numerous observers have considered Java over-populated since the early nineteenth century, and one wonders what

112

colonial officials may have thought after the census of 1930 (when the population was found to be 41.7 million) about the possibility of supporting almost double that number on Java by 1974'.[5]

Table 6.4

Role of economic sectors

	Labour force a in 1971 (millions)	Rate of growth % b (annual average) (1969-73)	Employment c elasticity
Agriculture	26.50	4.0	.2
Mining and quarrying	0.08	15.5	.1
Manufacturing	2.68	7.5	.1
Power and water	0.04	7.4	.4
Construction	0.68	22.7	.6
Services, etc.	4.12	2.4	
Trade, restaurants, etc.	4.26	n.a.	
Transport	0.95	13.8	.4
Other	1.97	n.a.	
Total	41.26	7.4	

a Labour force: *Statistik Indonesia 1974/75*, Biro Pusat Statistik Jakarta, Table III-1.
b Rate of growth: Table XIV -2.
c Employment elasticity: Table 26 of *Income Distribution Employment and Growth: a Case Study of Indonesia*, World Bank Staff Working Paper No. 212, 1975.

In principle if half of the Javanese went to live in Sumatra the population per sq. km. would rise to 109 from its current level of about 40 and the Javanese ratio would fall to 282—its level before 1930. Likewise there are vast uninhabited areas in Kalimantan, Sulawesi and Iryan Jaya. It is therefore understandable that transmigration should have had such a strong appeal in the Indonesian context; by providing agricultural employment in the unsettled areas of the other islands, the pressure on Javanese land resources and job opportunities may be reduced.

The 'push' from Java and the 'pull' to the other islands

In general, migration patterns will reflect relative changes in perceived economic opportunities in different regions or countries. This hypothesis assumes that, in equilibrium, the decision to migrate is triggered by changes in these perceptions. In other words, the decision to migrate will not be related to the level of the difference between these perceptions which will reflect the fact that people have preferences for different locations. If incomes in Sumatra are expected to be, say $100 more than in Java, the typical Javanese would decide whether this premium warranted his migration to Sumatra. If this differential were to increase, there would be more Javanese who considered it worthwhile leaving Java for Sumatra and migration would tend to take place. In equilibrium, the population will distribute itself on the basis of the expected income opportunities in the different regions. In practice, when the distribution of the population changes, this will affect relative expected incomes in which case the simultaneous determination of regional income and population distribution is fairly complex.

Intuitively the relative income hypothesis distinguishes between 'push' and 'pull' factors in the determination of migration. Thus for a given set of economic prospects in Sumatra, migration from Java to Sumatra would occur if prospects in Java deteriorated and had the effect of pushing people out of Java. Alternatively, for given economic prospects in Java, if prospects in Sumatra were to improve, migration from Java to Sumatra would occur on account of the increased 'pull' of Sumatra with respect to Java. In general the balance of these 'push' and 'pull' factors will be varying over time and subsequently the pattern of migration will be varying too.

Thus, in the natural order of events, if population growth in Java indeed had the effect of lowering economic prospects there relative to the prospects in Sumatra, net migration from Java to Sumatra would tend to take place. The volume of the migration would depend on a variety of economic and social factors. For example, Javanese close family ties are likely to inhibit the migratory response and there may also be a 'migratory trap' in the sense that many poor people may not be able to afford the relocation costs of migration and that if and as they become poorer they sink deeper into this trap, they fail to migrate. In general, however, migratory movements will reflect private individuals' perceptions of where the prospects are best in both economic and social terms and in this sense the Javanese population problem would tend to look after itself. This does not mean that per capita incomes will improve; when a given expansion in the population migrates from Java to Sumatra total per capita incomes in Indonesia must fall (unless capital investment increases sufficiently) because there are more mouths to feed, but Sumatran per capita incomes are likely to be depressed from what they otherwise would have been and Javanese per capita incomes improved. Instead it means that in general the increased population is likely to distribute itself in an efficient fashion.

The crucial question discussed below is whether or not directed transmigration is likely to add or detract from this efficiency in the context of local settlement. Alternatively, one has to query why the population in Indonesia is so unequally distributed in the first instance instead of assuming that this inequality might form the basis of a solution to the Javanese population problem. Unless one assumes that the Indonesians are not the best judges of where their own interests lie, one would have to conclude that the unequal population distribution reflects the fact that at the present time the net balance between the 'pull' factors to the other islands and the 'push' factors from Java is not sufficient to warrant net migration from Java to the other islands.

This argument may be put somewhat differently. If the economic prospects in Sumatera had been particularly strong, in particular if the land had shown promise that was consistent with the scarcity of capital in Indonesia, the volume of migration would have been as large as in those parts of Latin America where migration and land settlement on super marginal land has been particularly virulent. From an economic standpoint the geographical distribution of the population is most probably in equilbrium and the emptiness of many regions in Indonesia may be attributed to their poor economic prospects, or their need for large amounts of capital investment which in Indonesia is very scarce. Later we explore the possibility that the distribution of the population is inefficient and identify the legitimate grounds for the government to intervene in the land settlement process to improve it. Before that, however, consideration should be made whether the Javanese problem of land productivity might not be solved in ways more efficient than transmigration.

The macroeconomic context of transmigration

Introduction

Transmigration is usually seen to have two main roles, the alleviation of population pressure inside Java, Madura and Bali and the development of economic resources in the other islands of Indonesia. In addition, however, transmigration is sometimes intended to have political objectives in the unification and intermingling of the various social groups that comprise Indonesia and in the settlement of people along border areas for strategic purposes. At the present time the main objective of transmigration is most probably regarded as regional resource development since it is generally understood that transmigration cannot significantly alleviate the rate of growth of population in Java, Madura, and Bali. As to the political and social objectives many observers remark that transmigrants have generally kept to themselves. In particular the Javanese have not intermingled socially with the indigenous population and instead have evolved a 'Little Java' mentality instead of a spirit of national unity that was originally intended.

115

Our present purpose, however, is not to assess the social and cultural achievements of transmigration, nor to evaluate any economic contribution transmigration might have made in the past. Instead the discussion focuses on the legitimate role that transmigration might play in the future economic development of the country. This is particularly relevant since the main role of transmigration is seen to be that of economic development.

It should be stated from the outset that the discussion that follows is inevitably tentative for two main reasons. First, the constraints and trends in a process as complex as economic development are not generally understood in the Indonesian context. Secondly, the dearth of reliable data in Indonesia makes an empirical test of any hypothesis extremely difficult if not impossible. The chapter therefore addresses itself to issues rather than conclusions. Nevertheless, the discussion is suggestive of a broad strategy for economic development in which most probably transmigration has at best an insignificant role to play and at worst a negative role.

We begin by summarising the macroeconomic situation in Indonesia insofar as it is relevant to the main theme of the analysis which is to discuss the causes of Indonesia's economic backwardness. In identifying these causes we may hope to clarify the barriers to development whose removal could form the basis of a strategy for economic development.

National investment behaviour

A plausible benchmark in an assessment of the adequacy of aggregate investment behaviour is to consider whether or not investment has been sufficient to prevent average per capita incomes from declining. In 1973 for example, average income per capita was Rp 46,991 and net investment was Rp 880 billion (measured in 1973 prices). The population was estimated to have grown by 3.31 million in which case net investment per capita of this new population was Rp 265,861. To maintain average per capita incomes constant in the face of this additional population, national income must grow by Rp 155.54 billion (3.31 million x Rp 46,991).[6]

In a recent study on Indonesia the incremental capital output ratio was assumed to be about 3.1 and the incremental labour output ratio about 1.9.[7] In the long run population growth and work force growth will be almost perfectly correlated. On the basis of the incremental labour output ratio national income would increase by about 1.38 per cent or Rp 84 billion. The deficit of Rp 71.54 billion (155.54-84) would have to be made up by net capital formation. On the basis of the incremental capital output ratio net investment would have to be Rp 221.8 billion (or Rp 132,000 per capita in 1976 prices). In 1973 net investment was in fact Rp 880 billion in which case national income would be Rp 212.3 billion more than the figure required to maintain constant per capita incomes which on this basis would rise by Rp 1,644 or some 3.5 per cent.

This growth rate in average per capita income compares closely with actual experience in Indonesia, especially when technical progress is taken into consideration. The main conclusion would seem to be that in the recent past aggregate net investment has been sufficient to surpass the maintenance of constant per capita income. Expressed in 1976 dollars net investment must be about $1.1 billion at least to maintain constant per capita incomes. The table below shows that since 1969 this figure has always been exceeded and that the margin of the excess (or investment for per capita income growth) has been rising quite dramatically.

Table 6.5

Investment patterns

	1969	1970	1971	1972	1973	1974
				$ (1976 prices)		
Net investment per capita	9.6	13.9	18.3	27.7	28.8	32.5
Net investment per additional capita	447	566.7	709.7	1,093.8	1,121.2	1,264.7
Net investment (billions)	1.1	1.7	2.2	3.5	3.7	4.3 a

a Depreciation estimated at $1.7 billion.

Table 6.5 may also serve as a rough guideline for an appropriate capital expenditure figure in the context of project appraisal. The discussion above suggests that the investment required to provide new entrants into the labour force with the 1976 average family income is about $1,900. Alternatively, a project that cannot generate this income at a family investment figure of less than $1,900 is misallocating capital at a prima facie level. If all the net investment was directed into the creation of new jobs, Table 6.5 suggests that per capita investment should be about $1,400 (extrapolating the second row of the table to 1976) or about $7,000 for a family of five. Indeed, the figure could be higher than this (about $8,560 assuming the population is growing by about 2.1 per cent per annum) since the official estimates most probably overstate the rate of population growth. This investment figure assumes that all of net economic growth is embodied in new jobs. On the other hand, if investment is intended to improve existing per capita incomes, the average investment per capita (line one of the table) should be about

$36 per capita or $180 per family of five. These low figures reflect both the scarcity of capital in Indonesia and the general level of poverty.

Income distribution

Unfortunately there are no data on the distribution of income in Indonesia. However, the Socio-Economic Survey of 1969/70 tabulates the percentage of population by monthly per capita expenditure.

Table 6.6 concentrates on the expenditure of the lowest 40 per cent of those surveyed.

Table 6.6

Expenditure distribution per capita mid-1976$ a

Lowest:	1½%	10%	25%	42%
1969/70	26.5	44.2	66.4	88.5
End 1976	36.8	61.4	92.3	123.0

a *Survey Social Ekonomie Nasional 1969/70;* Biro Pusat Statistik, Jakarta 1973 Table 1 October 1969—April 1970 total Indonesia. Since the survey, prices have tripled as of mid-1976.

This table shows that in 1969/70 42 per cent of the population in Indonesia expended less than $88.5 per capita per annum and 10 per cent less than $44.2. One estimate of the poverty line (based on nutritional adequacy, housing and clothing) in Indonesia is about $90 per capita in 1976 prices. However, this assumes a diet based on rice which is expensive in terms of the provision of basic nutrients. In addition, the data upon which this calculation has been made are unreliable. The poverty line based on a cost minimisation approach to diet adequacy is approximately $60 per capita.[9] In 1969/70 about 42 per cent of the population were below the first poverty line and about 22 per cent below the second.

Since the survey was conducted, by the end of 1976, per capita income had most probably risen by about 39 per cent in real terms. The second row in Table 6.6 calculates the expenditures of the four subgroups under the assumption that the distribution of income has remained unaltered. On this assumption less than 25 per cent fall below the first poverty line and less than 10 per cent below the second. Thus over a period of seven years the poverty line has receded by about 15 percentage points. If this progress were to continue it would take less than five years to eliminate poverty using the $60 definition and about ten years to eliminate poverty on the basis of the $90 definition.

Table 6.7 below indicates that since 1970 (arbitrarily used as a base year) Indonesian prices have risen out of line with world prices (expressed in dollars) by a substantial margin. The import price index has been constructed out of the export prices of Indonesia's principal suppliers and the overseas consumer price index refers to Indonesia's export (nonoil) markets. [10] Since 1970, therefore, the Indonesian price level has risen by about 55 per cent over world prices. This divergence, however, has only become severe since 1973/74.

Table 6.7

Balance of payments indicators

	1970	1971	1972	1973	1974	1975	1976
Consumer prices (Rp)	100	104	111	146	205	244	287
Import prices ($)	100		107	136	182	184	195
Overseas consumer prices ($)	100		111	125	154	169	171
Change in reserves ($ millions)	38	27	397	233	685	-906	1,367

Under normal circumstances this would have resulted in a serious balance of payments problem. However, since 1974 the oil price hikes have been adding approximately $4 billion to the balance of payments per year. Prior to the oil price hikes the Indonesian balance of payments was broadly in equilibrium. The deficit in 1975 was largely attributable to the financial difficulties of Pertamina. Since then, however, the balance of payments has strengthened despite an anticipated capital account deficit in 1976 of about $2.2 billion. Thus, while the oil account has been adding about $4 billion to the balance of payments, the reserve flow has improved by only a fraction of this figure. Most probably a large part of the explanation may be attributed to the observation that since 1974 Indonesia's prices have fallen out of line with her competitors' prices.

The lag between the current account and relative prices is usually long, extending up to five years. Therefore, the nonoil account may well deteriorate over the next few years, and if the gap between Indonesia and world inflation continues to grow this development would be exacerbated. On this basis in 1978/79 Indonesia may well be faced with a balance of payments problem which it does not have at present.

Had the price of oil remained unchanged the rupiah would most probably have been devalued by now by about 50 per cent against the dollar. [11] The oil price hike has subsequently had the effect of eroding profit margins on the nonoil components of the balance of payments and generated a net deindustrialising effect on the economy as a whole. For example since 1973 rubber prices have risen by about 17 per cent on the world market while domestic prices have doubled. This implies a critical loss in relative profit margins in rubber production. In the short run rubber production would not be affected but the long run effects must be serious. This picture is typical of the majority of Indonesia's staple exports. A similar analysis applies to import substitution in Indonesia, especially in manufacturing where profit margins have been seriously eroded.

There is a very real danger therefore that the balance of payments benefits of the oil price hikes will indirectly have a deindustrialising effect on the economy as a whole through the obviation of any immediate pressure for a devaluation. If transmigration and similar projects are intended to release people from low productivity employment, it must seriously be considered whether the appropriate remedy lies in the microeconomic forum of project work or in the macroeconomic forum of exchange rate adjustment and related macroeconomic policies. It would most probably be more efficient to generate employment via the appropriate macroeconomic policies than via project work. Alternatively, more productive jobs could be created by establishing an appropriate exchange rate and at a lower cost than by project work. Attention must therefore be paid to the very real danger of pursuing transmigration as well as other microeconomic policies when the appropriate remedy is inherently macroeconomic.

Industrial policy

The relative importance of labour to capital in the production process will tend to reflect the relative advantages of labour to capital and in particular relative factor prices. In Indonesia it would seem that current industrial and labour policies discriminate against labour utilisation in favour of capital. In many cases, therefore, capital is used where otherwise labour might have been more efficient and aggregate employment potential is lower than it might otherwise have been. A recent study on Indonesian industry argues,[11]

> It is not absolutely clear which factors caused the failure of Indonesia's manufacturing industry to provide more employment. According to Boucherie's enquiries, one important factor may have been the present labour legislation (inherited from the pre-1965 period). In the pursuit of assuring job security, protecting workers against exploitation and improving general working conditions, the legislation makes it difficult and often virtually impossible for entrepreneurs to dismiss unneeded workers, it set

up minimum wage rates which are often in discordance with given productivity levels, it makes it expensive to use workers for overtime (more than 40 hours per week) and night shifts, and it limits the possibility of resorting to female employees. Thus, the labour legislation may reduce or even neutralise advantages which entrepreneurs in principle could derive from prevailing low wage rates. To the extent that entrepreneurs cannot circumvent these regulations (as is probably the case with large-scale and foreign firms), they are prone to adopt more capital-intensive methods of production than they otherwise would and to keep the pool of permanent employees as small as possible.

In addition to this the Foreign Investment Law (January 1967) and the Domestic Investment Law (November 1968) provide up to five years of tax holidays, accelerated depreciation, investment allowances, exemptions of duty on capital imports in many cases etc., all of which add up to a substantial encouragement to capital intensive methods. In addition, in many cases entrepreneurs can finance capital investment at subsidised and negative real interest rates which further boosts the bias in favour of capital intensive production methods.

As in the case of exchange rate policy, it must be asked to what extent the paucity of productive employment opportunities is related to industrial and labour policies as presently practiced and that the pre-occupation with employment creation at the microeconomic level of project implementation might be more gainfully applied at the macro level of redesigning these policies.

The mismatch hypothesis

An interesting hypothesis about Indonesia's economic backwardness is that there is a mismatch between existing production techniques, especially in manufacturing, and factor availabilities in Indonesia. On the whole manufacturing technologies have been developed in the industrialised countries and subsequently tend to be capital intensive. In poor countries such as Indonesia capital tends to be scarce and cheap unskilled labour in relative abundance. If manufacturing technologies are imported only a limited amount of labour will be absorbed given the shortage of capital since the technology will not match the indigenous factor availabilities.

The solution to the mismatch dilemma is either to modify the technology in order to match the factor availabilities or to modify the factor availabilities in order to match the technology. The former solution consists of inventing new technologies which is inherently difficult. The latter solution mainly consists of teaching skills to the labour force since an important aspect of the mismatch is the shortage of human capital. The long-term solution to the mismatch dilemma therefore leans heavily on education.

No doubt in Indonesia there is some degree of mismatch. Nevertheless, Donges et al remarked,

> Surprisingly, in view of the still low literacy rate, scarcity of skills in general seemed to be no bottleneck for the maintenance and/or expansion of industrial production. Local labour markets proved able to provide the enterprises with sufficiently skilled labourers. The most important sources of industrial skills seems to be both vocational and on-the-job training ... The only skills perceived to be scarce by the entrepreneurs are those related to supervisory personnel and middle management in very large plants (p.44).

In addition, 'The conclusion to be drawn ... is that labour markets in Indonesia are operating surprisingly efficiently in allocating labour in an economically appropriate way' (p.40). In general the study of Donges et al does not lend much support to the mismatch hypothesis. Their finding was that there is a reasonable and rational degree of substitutability between labour and capital.

Even if there is no general mismatch in certain cases there could be what might be called a wage-technology trap. This trap occurs where even with a subsistence wage it is cheaper to use capital rather than labour and because wages are by assumption at their subsistence level, they cannot fall any further to compete with capital. An example of this is the replacement of the ani-ani by the sickle that has occurred with the breakdown of agricultural involution in Java[13] where the more labour intensive ani-ani of harvesting can never compete with the sickle method.

Constraints to growth

Perhaps the most striking feature about the Indonesian economy is that despite an abundance of cheap labour it has failed to copy the prototypes of Taiwan, Korea, Japan, Hong Kong and other SE Asian countries where cheap labour formed the basis of economic growth with particular emphasis on the manufacturing sector. In view of what has been said above it would seem that labour is not a constraint to development and that other factors are in effect responsible for holding back the economic potential of the labour force.

Several contenders spring to mind. First, it seems generally recognised that the poor provision of infrastructure tends to impede economic progress. It is said that it costs more to transport goods from the other islands to Jakarta than from Tokyo to Jakarta, and farm or factory gate prices are sometimes only 30 per cent of market prices i.e. once the goods have been transported to their place of consumption. Very frequently therefore the manufacturer finds it difficult to take advantage of the cheap labour that is available since the costs of transporting both inputs and outputs are prohibitive. The provision of an effective transportation infrastructure is particularly important in a poor country such as Indonesia where the absence of an adequate or local market makes easy access to the world market particularly important.

A related constraint is the poor system of telecommunications which becomes particularly troublesome during work hours when it is needed most. Likewise the power grid is unreliable. Thus in many respects Indonesia lacks the basic infrastructure for development.

A further constraint is the practice of widespread corruption which has the effect of stifling economic initiative in an antisocial way and creating uncertainty where it would not naturally exist. Businessmen frequently find that they have to pay bribes to officials in order to obtain their goods from the customs or to obtain necessary licencing etc.

The intention in this section has not been to provide a full review of the constraints to growth in Indonesia. Nevertheless, there is a *prima facie* case that poor infrastructure is a major bottleneck in the growth process.

Strategy for growth and the role of transmigration

The foregoing arguments do not point to transmigration as a major component in Indonesian growth strategy. The basis of this strategy would be to formulate microeconomic policies within an appropriate macroeconomic policy framework. In particular the following items may be singled out.

(a) The exchange rate in an oil rich economy like Indonesia should ensure a sufficient degree of profitability to the production of exportables and import substitutes. At present this objective is not being achieved.

(b) Industrial and labour policy should be geared to the efficient use of Indonesia's factor endowments. At present these policies are contributing to an unnatural degree of capital intensity.

(c) Because capital is scarce it must be allocated with care and must guarantee a satisfactory rate of return to the economy as a whole. Accordingly, a fairly high test discount rate is appropriate—of the order of 18 per cent.[14] Projects which are expected to yield less than this in real terms would constitute a *prime facie* misallocation of scarce capital.

(d) Investment in infrastructure would be a priority insofar as poor infrastructure has been diagnosed as a constraint to growth.

This strategy would tend to maximize demand and minimize the barriers to the economic response to this demand. In turn employment and productivity would tend to be maximized and in the long term the role of manufacturing in the economy would be raised whereas in recent years it has been stagnant at about 9 per cent of GDP. Given the scarcity of unsettled fertile land and capital but an abundance of labour, agriculture will have to give way to manufacturing as the basis for economic growth in the future. Indonesia's chief asset is her labour which must be used to add value through international trade in manufacturing in the way that other land scarce prototypes have done in SE Asia.

In this context transmigration as it has been practiced in the past has amounted to an allocation of scarce capital in areas of limited and even submarginal agricultural potential with virtually no contribution to Indonesia's economic development. Moreover, in many cases the poverty of Java has been exported to various parts of the other islands to no social avail. In a real sense therefore, past investment in transmigration has most probably amounted to little more than investment in subsistence.

The longer term scarcity of agricultural potential in Sumatera is such that within a generation or so all the remaining 11.3 million ha of farmable land will be filled by natural population growth among the Sumaterans themselves (assuming holdings of about ¼ ha per capita of the rural population[15] and a population growth rate in line with the historic trend of 2.8 per cent per year). Thus the induced settlement of this land by transmigrants merely brings this date of land exhaustion forward. From this aspect too, transmigration would not be making any contribution to Indonesian economic development.

This suggests that if transmigration policies are to be continued agriculture is unlikely to be an appropriate mode within the context of Indonesia's development needs. Instead, industrial based transmigration might be more usefully explored. Nevertheless, it would seem that the thrust of government involvement in Indonesia's economic development should be in terms of the relief of the constraints to growth and the maintenance of appropriate macroeconomic policies.

Land settlement, the role of government and the design of transmigration projects

Introduction

Transmigration is a form of land settlement which entails an extensive degree of government involvement. The objective of this section is to determine the appropriate form of government involvement in transmigration on the basis of a plausible set of principles of land settlement and the allocation of capital. These are discussed under the heading 'Principles', and since the principles of capital allocation to be suggested are reasonably familiar, attention is focused on the more controversial subject of the principles and practice of land settlement. In this context examples of different forms of land settlement in various parts of the world will be presented in order to arrive at a set of land settlement principles that enjoy a reasonable degree of empirical support.

Under the heading 'Indonesian transmigration policy' these principles will be brought to bear on the design of transmigration projects. At all times the objective will be to allocate land, labour and capital in a way that is most advantageous to the Indonesians.

Two cardinal conditions for successful land settlement are identified. These are:

(a) The land must be supermarginal. Marginal or submarginal lands, or lands which can only be developed through the misallocation of capital are bound by definition to result in unsuccessful settlement.

(b) The settlers must be highly motivated. Pioneering is one of the most challenging of economic activities and only the most committed stand any chance of success.

These conditions are mutually re-enforcing; they stand or fall together. Good lands with unmotivated settlers, or highly motivated settlers on submarginal lands are unlikely to prove to be successful combinations.

A number of important but less crucial conditions for success may be identified. For example:

(a) Settlement should not be at vast distances beyond the frontier so that pioneer areas build on the economic strength of existing frontier areas.

(b) Settlers should be able to look forward to the establishment of their land tenure rights with a reasonable degree of certainty.

(c) The authorities should narrow the discrepancies between private and social settlement costs e.g. by building bridges, malarial control etc. in areas that otherwise show economic promise.

(d) The authorities should make capital available to the settlers in the event of capital market failure.

(e) Land and soil surveys should be made available by the relevant agencies so that information on areas of economic potential may be made known to the people of the inner islands.

From a practical point of view the processes of natural selection would be responsible for the best choice of settler. Almost by definition, the unspontaneous settler who prefers the more organised form of government settlement schemes tends to be less than highly motivated. These conditions imply that the private or unassisted model should form the basis of land settlement, and that the authorities should play an active role in easing the land settlement process and increasing its chances of success rather than actually initiating it.

In many aspects the principal conditions for land settlement failure are the obverse of the conditions for success. From a political point of view the chances of failure tend to compound themselves in situations where the authorities choose pioneers from overcrowded areas or areas where the economic potential seems to be exhausted, and settles them in submarginal lands which are empty by virtue of their submarginality.

In the light of the land reviews, this danger of failure is very real in Indonesia. Indeed, the poor quality of the land in the other islands is responsible for much of the government's involvement in transmigration since the authorities feel they have to push for settlement where it would otherwise not naturally take place by providing various artificial stimuli to land settlement. The Indonesian scene differs fundamentally and depressingly from the Latin American situation where much of the unsettled land is supermarginal and where the problems that confront the authorities are altogether different. There the problem is not how can the authorities generate land settlement, but how can they best assist the natural dynamism towards land settlement that is driven by an abundance of good land.

Thus, at first sight it may seem that the Indonesian population is inefficiently distributed. In a narrow geographical sense this is of course true; but in terms of the resource endowment of the country both with regard to land potential and capital availability, it is likely that the present aggregative population distribution is in equilibrium. Alternatively, the first question to be raised on observing unpopulated areas is why this is the case. Usually the answer is that the land is of poor quality and that its costs of development are too high. The evacuation of people from overcrowded areas of the inner islands to relatively infertile, unpopulated areas in the other islands is at best postponing a real problem in an inefficient fashion while being counterproductive with regard to the economic development of the country and, at worst, it could be harmful to both the short term and long term aspirations of the very people that such a well meaning policy was ostensibly designed to foster.

Principles

Basic principles

The profit motive would tend to insure that the marginal productivity of land in different areas of the same region would be related. If, for example, the marginal productivity of land were higher in area B than in area A, farmers would be tempted to reallocate their work in favour of area B in order to take advantage of the higher profit prospects there. The marginal productivity of land in area B would fall and it would tend to rise in area A. In the limit, i.e. if there were no relocation and adjustment costs, and if farmers regarded working in the two areas as perfect substitutes, agricultural equilibrium would be restored when the marginal productivities of land were equated. Thus if for example area B enjoyed a superior agricultural climate to area A, the *ex post* marginal productivities of land would be the same although area B would be more heavily farmed than area A.

In practice this limit is unlikely to prevail for a number of reasons. If area B is located at a considerable distance from area A, the costs of relocation would tend to generate a differential between the respective marginal productivities since these costs would in part make it unprofitable for farmers to arbitrage away the differential in marginal land productivities. Secondly, if farmers have a preference for working in say area A (on account of a more enjoyable climate, family ties, etc.) the marginal productivity of land in A will tend to be below the marginal productivity of land in B since the land in A will be relatively overworked. Thirdly, if agriculture in area B is riskier than in area A on account of say a less reliable climate farmers will prefer to operate in area B and the marginal productivity of land will be subsequently greater in B than in A.

While marginal land productivities might differ at any point in time, they will tend to be related through time. If agricultural equilibrium initially prevails and there is an exogenous increase in the marginal productivity of land in area B, farmers will be motivated to some degree to increase their efforts in area B. This will cause the marginal productivity of land in A to rise in sympathy with the initial exogenous increase in area B. These relationships can be expected to prevail in the long run. In the short run there may be substantial divergencies between marginal productivities of agricultural land which occur during the adjustment process. For the present, however, our concern is with the long run or the trend in agricultural development in land settlement where these short term effects can be ignored.

Land settlement

This marginal productivity theory of land use may be extended into a theory of land settlement. New land might be settled for three main reasons in this neoclassical context. First, as the population grows, lands which are currently marginal will come under cultivation via the familiar Malthusian dynamic. The shape of the land settlement frontier would depend on the distribution of the natural qualities of the land. If this distribution is fairly uniform the frontier would be correspondingly uniform too. An uneven distribution on the other hand would lead to a jagged frontier. At all points on the frontier the marginal productivity of the land would be related along the lines described in the previous section.

Secondly, lands which are currently submarginal might be settled on account of technological improvements which render them supermarginal. For example, arid areas which are irrigated would come under cultivation. Indeed, technological improvements might change the level of the margin and lands which were initially above the old margin might now be below the new margin and will subsequently go out of cultivation.

Thirdly, land is frequently unsettled due to uncertainty about its agricultural potential. Subsequently, new information about land beyond the frontier would tend to change the pattern of land settlement. In this context the role of the pioneer is crucial. However, first a simple model of pioneering is developed.

A model of pioneering

Land pioneering is intrinsically hazardous but potentially rewarding. The established farmer has to make a comparison between the reasonably steady income that he presently obtains and the relatively uncertain income that he might obtain as a pioneer. On the whole, people are highly risk averse, preferring the bird in the hand to the two in the bush. Indeed, the majority of us act on the basis of a 'safety first' principle where the risk of disaster is given a weighting which is proportionally larger than the risk of success. We all dream of success but disaster cannot be afforded and safety must come first.

The 'safety first' principle for the most part would tend to restrain the pioneering spirit. However, each farmer will make his own subjective calculation and those who on balance consider their expectations as a pioneer to be sufficiently high relative to their current expectations will elect to move beyond the frontier. It will be in the nature of things that pioneers will be few since the 'safety first' principle will dominate the thinking of the vast majority of farmers.

This model lends itself to the conclusion that pioneers are likely to be people who can afford to take large risks e.g. because they have alternative livelihoods inside the frontier, or because they are already at risk inside the frontier e.g. people whose land inheritance is likely to reduce the size of individual land holdings.

Dynamics of pioneering

Once the pioneers have established themselves the risks as perceived by the farmer inside the frontier diminish assuming the lands that have been pioneered have economic potential. Most probably the perceived risk falls slowly but eventually and as the news filters through the assessment of risk could eventually fall dramatically. Initially, therefore, secondary settlement might be small, but eventually the number of secondary settlers would tend to swell as the drop in perceived risk disturbs their equilibrium land settlement position.

This dynamic raises an important issue of policy since the pioneers play an important social role in reducing perceived risk which is effectively distorting the patterns of land settlement from its Pareto-optimal allocation. A subsidy that encouraged successful pioneering would generate social benefits in the form of a more favourable pattern of land settlement. However, great care would be required to avoid the danger of making pioneering a soft option since *ex ante* the perceived risks are realistic and those that are less than highly motivated are unlikely to become successful pioneers.

A related policy issue is that the authorities should seek to reduce perceived risk by conducting soil and topographical surveys in prospective pioneer areas. While privately these costs are high, socially they are quite low. Indeed, in many cases this would be the only legitimate involvement of government in the initial processes of land settlement.

If the newly pioneered areas are sufficiently supermarginal some of the originally settled areas could become obsolescent since the concept of the margin would rise. Thus it is possible for the frontier to shift out in one direction but to move back in another.

Externalities and the role of government

The process of land settlement implied by the pioneer augmented neo-classical model might be held up by a variety of natural causes which create divergences between the private and social rates of return to land settlement. For example, land which is cut off by a river or a canyon will have a high private entry cost but a much lower social entry cost since for society as a whole the cost of a bridge is low but for the individual is most probably prohibitive. Otherwise viable areas which are unsettled on account of a high divergence between private and social entry costs could be settled if the authorities sought to narrow such natural market imperfections by selectively establishing access points into areas of land settlement potential.

Apart from mapping etc. and the traditional role of maintaining law and order in newly settled areas the legitimate role of government in the pioneering process should be confined to investment infrastructure whose purpose is to narrow the divergence between private and social costs of settlement since this will generate legitimate land settlement where otherwise it would not have occurred. As for the rest, pioneering and land settlement should be left to market forces where the individual who unaided and unsponsored takes his life into his own hands is most likely to succeed.

This argument should be contrasted with the often voiced proposition that land settlement is too socially important to be left to the ebbs and flows of market forces and that instead land settlement should be the government's comprehensive responsibility. In particular it is argued that land settlement is an aspect of land reform which is designed to redistribute land in favour of the landless. However, given the extremely high degree of motivation required for pioneering and land settlement it would seem inappropriate to use land settlement as an instrument of redistributive policies. Indeed, the high risks of failure inherent in such policies most probably work against the best interests of the members of those target groups that are selected by the government to be pioneers. Once an area has been pioneered by naturally and spontaneously motivated settlers the authorities may face the political challenge of land distribution. Obviously, fear of expropriation for such purposes, especially in the context of the 'safety first' principle could act as a serious damper on land settlement.

The general principle of government involvement implicitly assumes that the authorities know better than the market where economic prospects lie and consider themselves more capable than those who would spontaneously choose to become pioneers at successfully settling an area. If anything, civil servants are likely to make unrealistic assessments of risk since unlike the spontaneous settler they risk the taxpayer's money rather than their own resources and for related reasons would be less motivated to make projects succeed. Whereas the private individual puts safety first, the civil servant is often motivated unduly to discount safety since at no stage does he risk his own life and resources.

It may happen that the pattern of land settlement is distorted by fears of government confiscation or partial appropriation of land which is successfully settled. In this case land would not be settled even though it would have been economically viable, and these fears set up a counter-productive divergence between social and private risk. Some observers believe this to be the case in Indonesia where the expropriation of private estates during the Sukarno era has firghtened private investors from developing estates in the other islands. Under these circumstances the authorities have two fundamental choices in political economy. The first is that they should invest where the private sector has been discouraged by their predecessors. However, this option may further discourage the development of the private sector and misallocate capital long the lines already discussed. The second is to foster an atmosphere in which the private sector will feel more confident and to remove the constraints which the authorities have previously imposed on private investment behaviour. In repairing damages in the past the second approach would be preferable, but the time horizons may be long.

The allocation of capital

The principles of capital allocation are analogous to the principles of land allocation and efficiency would be achieved when capital flows to where its rewards are highest. Here too the market itself is likely to be the best judge of where capital will serve its most useful purpose.

In many developing countries, however, capital markets are imperfect in the sense that the institutions do not exist to allocate capital in an efficient manner. Often access to banks does not exist and private projects fail to be implemented because of an unnatural absence of capital. Malfunction of the capital market is likely to occur where the processes of financial intermediation are themselves government controlled and where officials are sluggish in establishing financial intermediation especially in the more remote areas where the private financier might be tempted to move in. Whatever the cause of capital market failure, the authorities would be justified in encouraging financial intermediation either directly by the provision of capital or indirectly by reorganising the private capital market.

In the context of land settlement capital should in general be raised privately by the settlers themselves at the going rate of interest. If interest rates are too high for prospective settlers this is a sign of capital scarcity in which case the allocation of capital for land settlement would be inefficient and there would be no case for subsidised interest rates. If the capital market is imperfect in the sense that prospective settlers feel they can cover commercial interest rates but do not have access to the market it would be legitimate for the authorities to offer settlers the capital at the going commercial rate of interest. To offer the capital in the form of a grant or at a subsidised rate of interest, i.e. at the taxpayer's expense, would only be legitimate if society as a whole were to benefit from the use of the capital.

For example, if there is no divergence between economic and private rates of return there should be no difference between the rate of interest the settler pays and the market rate of interest. If the social or economic return is above the private return, the settler should pay a subsidised interest rate that equates the social rate of return with the opportunity cost on capital. This is illustrated in Figure 6.1 where it is assumed that as the capital stock rises the return on capital falls. AB is the private return schedule and AC is the schedule with regard to the social rate of return on capital. In other words the social return is assessed to be always greater than the private return. Oa denotes the private opportunity cost of capital which is assumed for simplicity to be the same as the social opportunity cost of capital. The investor will subsequently invest Od, but the social rate of return will be dc. To equate the social rate of return with social opportunity cost of capital, the private rate of interest must be reduced to Og so that Oe is invested and the social rate or return falls to ef = Oa.[16]

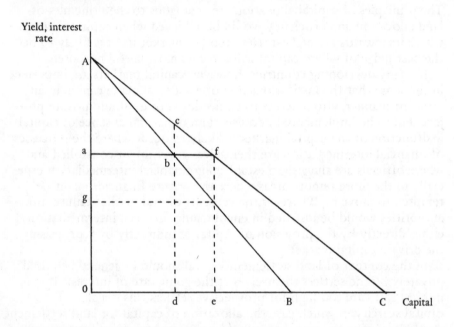

Figure 6.1 The social rate of return on capital

The optimal interest rate subsidy is therefore ga. If the private return is always above the social return, the argument is reversed and a punitive interest charge would be desirable. If therefore the social rate of return is equal to the rate of interest but the private rate of return is zero the optimal subsidy would require that no interest be paid. If the private rate of return is negative under the same circumstances the optimal

132

subsidy would require that some of the principal be retained by the investor. In the limit the optimal subsidy would take the form of a grant. Alternatively, the provision of subsidised credit or grants has the effect of redistributing income to the recipients in the absense of off-setting external social economies.

In this connection, it is sometimes argued that if interest collection costs are high in relation to the rate of interest, the loan should be treated as a grant. For example, if the rate of interest is 10 per cent but it costs the equivalent of 10 per cent to collect the interest, the loan should be made over as a grant. In general, this argument is unreasonable since the lender would obviously be at a loss and society not compensated for the subsidy involved. The appropriate interest charge would be 20 per cent since the costs of capital provision are no different to the costs of providing any other resource or service. The provision of grants where loans are otherwise desirable redistributes income in an inefficient way.

Practice

Effect of government intervention on land settlement

The main focus of this chapter is to assess the appropriate role of government in the process of land settlement. In particular are there any general principles which enjoy empirical support and which would determine the balance between public and privately sponsored land settlement? The main deductions of the previous section might be summarised as follows:

(a) Land will be settled in accordance with its marginal productivity.

(b) Pioneers are likely to be highly motivated people who can afford to take large risks.

(c) Land settlement is best left to the private sector.

(d) Government involvement in land settlement is likely to reduce the chances of success because of the difficulties in choosing pioneers and because of the potential downward bias in the assessment of risk.

(e) The role of government should be limited to providing infra-structure that narrows the gap between private and social settlement costs in an efficient way.

(f) In general the authorities should supply credit and not grants to viable settlers. If the capital market is imperfect subsidies should only be made available where external economics are generated.

(g) The authorities should ensure satisfactory land titling and
perform the traditional functions of government such as the
maintenance of law and order in newly settled areas. They
should naturally supply those resources over which they may
effectively have control such as fertilizer, extension services,
etc.

In the present context the most important points are (c) and (d)
which as empirical propositions are testable in principle. While a world-
wide study of these hypotheses would inevitably be formidable and
beyond the scope of this chapter, the limited evidence that is available
would seem to provide sufficiently strong support for them as to be of
general applicability.

Perhaps the most influential study is that of Michael Nelson[17] based
on 24 land settlement projects in the humid tropics of Latin America.
His main conclusions are worth quoting verbatim:

> But few spheres of economic development have a history of, or
> reputation for, failure to match that of government-sponsored
> colonisation in humid tropical zones. Horror stories abound
> about expensive ventures that resulted in colonies where few
> if any settlers remained after several years ... The evidence is
> irrefutable, and failure can be attributed only to the institutions
> responsible for selecting the area and the colonists, planning
> and executing the development programme, and subsequently
> maintaining or abandoning the infrastructure and services in
> the region. (p.265)

Furthermore, there is a conflict between the spirit of pioneering and
the prepackaged nature of government directed land settlement.

> Deliberate programmes for settler recruitment have constituted
> a failure element; self reliant pioneer colonists are not necessa-
> rily attracted by the programmes, and the executive agency
> tends to be drawn into expensive paternalistic operations.
> (p.273)

The wrong settlers are chosen. Indeed, the only reliable selection procedure would seem to be that of nature herself.

Care should be taken in interpreting these observations. The crucial
test is not whether government directed ventures have failed, but whether
there was a significant incidence of failure relative to the unassisted
ventures on supermarginal lands. Failure on submarginal lands is of
course to be expected and it is possible that governments might be
tempted to settle submarginal lands i.e. where the unassisted settler does
not wish to go. Nelson suggests that the incidence of failure was indeed
significant.

In all of these cases, as in the directed pioneer projects, viable agriculture proved to be possible. The success or failure of the projects depended on the institutional conditions that guided the proportions of the production factors in the exploitation of the regions. The directed projects were saddled with high public expenditures and a rigid design based on information that could not be as accurate as assumed without excessive expenditures for studies on hydrology, sociology, anthropology, soils, and so on. Spontaneous pioneer settlement was not burdened by high overheads, and projects launched in the consolidation phase had the benefit of a considerable accumulation of information on the factors listed above. (p.275)

In other words, government directed settlement projects have tended to fail for at least three main reasons:

(a) the difficulties inherent in selecting pioneers;

(b) the lack of flexibility inherent in organised settlement;

(c) underestimate of risks given the information base.

In her comparative study of unassisted and government directed settlers in the Philippines, Horakova[18] notes that the spontaneous settlers are more self reliant and that their government sponsored counterparts tended to pass over the responsibility for their livelihoods to the government.

In Africa too, Chambers' study of directed settlement[19] suggests that the government sponsored approach to land settlement has been unsatisfactory from the points of view of selection, technique and organisation. Here the main problem was that the 'pioneers' who were selected seemed to regard settlement as a form of social welfare and failed to insinuate themselves into the spirit of the various projects. A similar theme is developed by Farmer in the case of Sri Lanka and India.[20] As far as selection and land use in particular are concerned, however, Farmer is doubtful of the economic viability of the Sri Lanka projects. Nevertheless (pp.359-374) he goes on to discount the private settlement model as impractical in Sri Lanka and while he recommends a multifaceted approach to land settlement based on different sizes of land holdings, he envisages a strengthening and improvement of existing methods of directed settlement. Like Gunnar Myrdal, in his 'Asian Drama', Farmer's reaction to a failure of planning is to recommend a yet stronger form of planning.

Dozier[21] too notes that 'Adequate empirical evidence exists that not even the most bountiful combination of other conditions can be effective without the proper kind of colonists to go with them', (p.198) and that it will seem that 'A real danger appears in overproviding and overplanning for the colonist to the extent that independence and incentive disappear or never develop'. (p.206) In other words there is an inherent conflict between formal selection procedures which tend to attract dependent people and the needs of the land beyond the frontier which are for independent and highly motivated pioneers.

There have been several comparative studies of the economic success of unassisted and directed settlements. Apart from Nelson's results which indicate that the private and unassisted settler is more likely to succeed (p.264), Dozier notes that '... we find examples of spontaneous colonists whose returns are considerably higher than those of neighboring colonists on direct projects in the same tropical forest setting'. (p.215) Likewise, for the Philippines Horokova shows that the unassisted settlers have outperformed the assisted settlers on the basis of a variety of different economic and social criteria, and Fitzgerald reports for Kalimantan that[22]

> Field evidence suggests very strongly that the most successful settlers are those pioneering largely as a result of their own initiative and individual decisions ... The least successful pioneers would seem to be government sponsored ...

Also the recent unpublished work of Gloria Davies suggests that in Central Sulawesi the most successful transmigrants were unassisted Balinese migrants whereas the sponsored Javanese transmigrant settlements for the most part ended up in disaster.

Most students of the Malaysian land settlement policy agree that while the highly directed FELDA has been a political success[23] it has been very expensive in economic terms and Wafa has argued that the[24] less capital intensive and more spontaneous Kelantan State Land Development Authority has deployed capital more economically than the management oriented FELDA scheme. In other words the higher yields of FELDA (roughly 55 per cent higher than KSLDA) obtained through greater inputs have not generated a new social surplus. By extensive capital investment FELDA has virtually taken the risk out of land settlement in a monocultural context in which case the choice of settler has been less crucial. However, many feel that the costs have been too high both absolutely and relative to alternative settlement methods.

The role of government

With the exception of Farmer, the students of land settlements surveyed suggest that government direction is inimical to land settlement and would recommend a more restricted role for government. However, it is worth noting that Farmer's evidence does not conflict with the general trend of the other evidence. In addition, it should be recalled that in the US the West was settled with the minimum of government involvement. Indeed, the model has for time immemorial been the universal basis for land colonisation (with the exception of penal colonies and exiles).

This does not imply that government has no role at all to play in land settlement; merely that its role should be suitably defined. Nelson concludes:

> This suggests the diversion of resources to activities that are less susceptible to uncertainties than the fragile socioeconomic experiments in the directed transfer of population to the tropical land frontier. The alternative lies in more emphasis on services to spontaneous settlement in the consolidation or growth state, or where pioneer colonisation is desired, on orienting programmes to penetration roads or private subdivisions. (pp.267-8)

In particular Nelson regards highway construction as a crucial role for government: 'If a single element is to be isolated as the prerequisite to success in new land development, it must be highways'. (p.271) For highways break down the divergence between private and social costs of settlement in two important respects. First they directly facilitate the penetration of new areas. Secondly, they provide the all important linkages to existing markets and sources of supply. In the absence of these linkages to markets the costs of transportation which may be very high would seriously limit the potential for land settlement.

In this connection both Nelson (p.265) and Dozier (p.197) remark that contiguous land settlement is likely to be more successful than if land is pioneered at vast distances from the existing frontier. Inevitably, transportation costs are likely to be lower in areas contiguous to the frontier than in remote enclaves that lie deep in the jungle. Also there is some evidence which suggests that pioneers from contiguous areas are likely to be more successful than settlers who originate from areas that are remote from the new settlement areas. Local pioneers will be more familiar with the land beyond the frontier than their more distant counterparts and in these areas will be at a distinct advantage.

The traditional role of government of maintaining law and order is of special importance in the context of market oriented land settlement which in the nature of things will almost inevitably involve conflicts between pioneers over land rights and related issues. A failure in this function could lead to disaster as in the case of, for example, Alto Ture in Brazil where settlement along a new highway degenerated into a chaos of land grabbing. The risks of pioneering are great enough without the additional burden of risk about titling.

Indonesian transmigration policy

The historical context

The history of transmigration in Indonesia shows that there has been continuous experimentation with various forms of government involvement in transmigration. During the 1930s this involvement was small under the Bawon system relative to the experimental period of 1905-31. Since the 1950s the pendulum has swung the other way and currently the involvement of government is as high as it has ever been before. However, it is worth noting as Pelzer points out[25] that the original Dutch idea in 1903 was for transmigration to follow an unassisted rather than a sponsored model, however, with the authorities sponsoring some initial settlement in selected areas.

It is also worth noting that transmigrants constitute about 40 per cent of total net life time out migration from Java and Bali whereas for the world only 25 per cent of land settlement is government sponsored. However, not all migrants are involved in land settlement and not all transmigrants are fully sponsored by the government. Nevertheless, it would seem that while the relative involvement of the Indonesian government in migration has been high, in absolute terms there are still more people who migrate on an unassisted basis than people who migrate with various forms of government assistance. In other words, there exists in Indonesia a significant basis for free market settlement.

Furthermore it must be asked whether the sponsored transmigrants would not have otherwise migrated on an unassisted basis. In the limit, by sponsoring migration the authorities might not be generating any net migration at all for two reasons. First, the transmigrants might in any case have gone on an unassisted basis. Secondly, the transmigrants might be using up the opportunities which would otherwise have attracted the unassisted migrants. A further possibility is that new migration would be reduced if the volume of unassisted migrants were to fall by more than the net increase in the volume of transmigrants, e.g. on account of additional risk perceived by the potential unassisted migrants. It is clear therefore that the macroeconomic contribution of transmigration policies must be less than its microeconomic or direct contribution.

A related issue is the policy of limiting the size of land holdings which in principle must sap migration potential. It is inevitable that the traditional 2-5 ha plot in the relatively unfertile other islands and the limited income that it can generate will not be sufficient to attract the successful farmers who perhaps by virtue of their success are most likely to succeed as pioneers. Instead this policy will tend to attract less motivated people who think that they are getting something for nothing rather than people who are motivated to make something of nothing. In this connection, there is an obvious danger that the grant package will attract people for the sake of the provision of subsistence and maintenance. This is particularly the case in a society where because of extreme poverty, discount rates are high and where what matters most is for the family to get by for the next 12-18 months and to tackle what is in store thereafter when the time comes.[26] Indeed, there is evidence to suggest that many Javanese regard transmigration as a form of charity that bears all the stigma and humiliation of the poorhouse. In the light of what has been argued in the previous section it is unlikely that this policy will be a basis for successful land settlement and migration.

Design in transmigration

The foregoing arguments would suggest the following general principles for project design in transmigration.

(a) The basis for land settlement and transmigration should be market oriented rather than management oriented.

(b) There should be no direct or indirect discrimination against settlers both by income class and geographical origin. This requires a homesteading policy with a considerably less restricted land ceiling than is currently practiced.

(c) The government should identify areas which have economic potential, carry out soils surveys, etc. and publicise the results as far as possible.

(d) They should identify areas where it seems that there is divergence between private and social settlement costs and provide the infrastructure (mainly roads and bridges) which would narrow this divergence in these areas which otherwise show signs of economic promise.

(e) If the capital market is imperfect they should provide credit on an economic basis and at unsubsidised interest rates unless the settlers are providing the rest of society with indirect economic advantages, e.g. improved terms of trade, etc. Grants would be economically and socially inefficient.

(f) Land settlement is an unsuitable medium for income redistribution policies given its inherent hazards.

(g) Land tenure rights should be unambiguous and society should be confident about their implementation. This is particularly important given that pioneering involves enough unavoidable risks.

(h) Once settlers have proved that they can establish themselves the government should provide social infrastructure such as local roads, schools, etc. on the basis of orthodox principles of public finance. They should also organise land titlings, extension services and provide those resources over which they happen to have control, e.g. fertilizers.

(i) The settlers should be free to determine what they consider to be an appropriate economic system for their land. There should be no political prejudgment on this system.

These broad principles are designed to permit settlers to get on with the job and for the authorities to help them in a legitimate fashion. However, they imply a considerable departure from current policies in Indonesia, while at the same time converging on a growing consensus about the role of the authorities in transmigration and land settlement policies elsewhere, e.g. INCORA in Columbia.

The political economy of transmigration

Past experience in various parts of the world emphasises the highly political nature of land settlement and the movements of peoples. No attempt will be made here to discuss the politics of land settlement other than to observe that there is no endemic reason why land settlement should inevitably fall under government control and sponsorship. Instead our remarks are directed at the economic interest that various vested interests might have in the politics of transmigration.

In the Indonesian case most probably the high degree of government control is largely attributable to the direct economic interests that civil servants have in the bureaucratisation of land settlement and transmigration (as well as other areas too). The profits from corruption inevitably favour a political economy of extensive government involvement, and the administration has the power to pursue its own interests. At the other end of the bureaucracy, the so called beneficiaries of transmigration are politically powerless since they are dependent on the favours of the civil servants who are after all transferring resources to them from the community at large. Such a system is inherently prone to abuse and the result is usually stagnation rather than economic and social development.

A second important factor behind the high degree of government involvement is the poor quality of the land in the other islands that is available for transmigration. In Latin America and especially Brazil where there is an abundance of prospective supermarginal land, land settlement does not need to be pushed since through the dynamics of the marginal productivity theory it happens naturally. By contrast in Indonesia the unsettled land or alternatively the lands that are still under shifting cultivation are submarginal (the reason why they are empty in the first place) given the scarcity of capital and in accordance with the marginal productivity theory land settlement and related migration are virtually absent. In this situation the authorities are politically tempted to provide artificial stimuli to land settlement through the provision of subsidies and an inefficient allocation of capital to land settlement where the economic rates of return are unduly low.

The fear is that if the authorities pursued a market oriented land settlement policy, there would be little or no transmigration. This would only happen if the land itself did not justify it and as previously observed the withdrawal of the authorities from land settlement and transmigration could act as a stimulus. If it did happen, the reality would have to be accepted. However, if such basic realities are not accepted serious economic development cannot begin.

Notes

1   The contents of this chapter are based on information available during the first half of 1977.

2   See W. L. Collier, Soentoro, Gunawan Wiradi, and Makali 'Agricultural Technology and Institutional Change in Java'. *Food Research Institute Studies, volume XIII, no. 2,* 1974; Food Research Institute, Stanford University, Stanford, California.

3   This elasticity relates to the percentage increase in employment associated with a 1 per cent increase in output.

4   See G. Jones, 'What do we know about the labour force in Indonesia?', *Majalah Demografi,* December 1974, Table 18.

5   B. White 'Population, Involution and Employment in Rural Java', *Development and Change,* Vol. 7, 1976, p.268.

6   These calculations are based on Table XV.3, *Statistik Indonesia 1974-5 Biro Pusat Statistic,* Jakarta, December 1975 and *International Financial Statistics,* IMF, December 1976, p.192.

7   See *Income Distribution, Employment and Growth: a Case Study of Indonesia,* World Bank Staff Working Paper No. 212 August 1975, Appendix IV page 7.

8   If an investment of $1,900 is to produce an average family income of about $1,150, a very high test discount rate on capital is implied.

9   Chapter 5.

10   The price indices are weighted average of the Industrial Countries and other Asia prices as published in the *International Financial Statistics* (IMF). In the case of import prices the weights are 50:50 and in the case of export prices 30:70. The figures for 1976 are naturally estimates based on mid-1976 values.

11   Since 1971 the effective exchange rate for the rupiah has been devalued by roughly 22 per cent.

12   See J. B. Donges, B. Stecher and F. Wolter *Industrial Development*

Policies for Indonesia, J. C. Mohr (Paul Siebeck), Tubingen 1974, p.16.

13   See W. L. Collier, Soentoro, Gunawan Wiradi and Makali 'Agricultural Technology and Institutional Change in Java', in *Food Research Institute Studies* Vol. XIII, No. 2, 1974, Stanford University, Stanford, California.

14   See Donges et al., op.cit., p.58, where Papanek suggests a test discount rate in the region of 15-20 per cent.

15   In 1973, 5.11 million ha of Sumatera land was under cultivation at a time when the rural population was about 20 million. If, in future, farm size holdings average 5 ha, the land would be filled by about 1990.

16   At this sectoral level it is reasonable to assume that the supply of capital is perfectly elastic. For the economy as a whole this would of course not be realistic.

17   M. Nelson, *The Development of Tropical Lands; Policy Issues in Latin America.* The John Hopkins University Press, Baltimore, and London, 1973.

18   Eva Horakova, *Problems of Filipino Settlers,* Occasional Paper No. 4, Institute of Southeast Asian Studies, Singapore.

19   Robert Chambers, *Settlement Schemes in Tropical Africa,* New York, Praeger, 1969.

20   B. H. Farmer, *Pioneer Peasant Colonisation in Ceylon,* Oxford University Press, London, 1957. Also, *Agriculture Colonisation in India Since Independence,* Oxford University Press, London, 1974.

21   Craig L. Dozier, *Land Development Colonisation in Latin America,* Frederick A. Praeger, New York, 1969.

22   Dennis P. Fitzgerald, 'Pioneer Settlement in Southern and East Kalimantan'.

23   See Colin MacAndrews, *Mobility and Modernisation: a Study of the Malaysian Federal Land Development Authority and its Role in Modernising the Rural Malay,* PhD Thesis at MIT, 1976.

24   S. H. Wafa, *Land Development Strategies in Malaysia: an Empirical Study,* PhD Thesis, Stanford University, 1972.

25   Karl J. Pelzer, *Pioneer Settlement in the Asiatic Tropics,* American Geographical Society Special Publication No. 29, 1945, p.191.

26   See D. H. Penny and J. Price Gittinger 'Economics and Indonesia Agricultural Development in *Indonesia: Resources and their Technological Development,* H. W. Beers (ed), The University Press of Kentucky, Lexington, 1970, p.265.

7 Transmigration and Indonesian economic development

Historical perspectives

Records show that concern about the overpopulation of Java dates back at least as far as the first part of the nineteenth century. The fear has always been that population growth in Java would outstrip the indigenous resource availability and that starvation would be inevitable unless some solution were found. One hundred and fifty years later, politicians and social scientists are still grappling with the same problem which is apparently tending to recede further into the future with an almost embarrassing sense of relief to those who have failed to find a solution comprehensive enough to match the apparent enormity of the problem of Javanese overcrowding.

'... one wonders what colonial officials may have thought after the census of 1930 (when the population was found to be 41.7 million) about the possibility of supporting almost double that number on Java by 1974'.[1] No doubt the threat of impending social disaster on account of population pressure was as real to some in 1930 as it is to others today. Unfortunately, absence of data does not enable us to determine whether the Javanese have been getting richer or poorer over the long term, although it is clear enough that the doom foreseen by previous generations of certain students of Java has not materialised. Indeed, a recent survey in Java indicates[2] that only 9 per cent of respondents thought that living conditions in Java have deteriorated over the previous generation, whereas 62 per cent thought they had improved. Incidentally, the same survey showed that only 4 per cent expected Javanese prospects to deteriorate, whereas 76 per cent thought they would improve. In addition, GDP per capita in Java has recently been growing annually by about 4.2 per cent and while as with any other economy, economic development may harm the prospects of those whose activities have become obsolescent through the application of superior technologies, the vast majority of the Javanese appear to be getting better off, and believe that their prospects are likely to improve in the future.

While the causes of this secular improvement have not been fully studied, one deduction is clear; 70 years of transmigration have contributed little if anything to this improvement. During this period there have been on average no more than 13,500 official transmigrants per year, or as much as the population growth in Java in less than 72 hours. All the evidence suggests that regardless of the apparent pressure on the land, productivity on Java has increased despite the virtual doubling of the population in less than 50 years. These observations are not intended to convey that all is well on Java. Rather they suggest that all is not as bad as some people make out, and subsequently that there is no justification for embarking on risky development strategies such as transmigration, where the argument has been that the threat of mass poverty in Java makes higher risk strategies worthy of practical consideration. In this context, as will be argued later, there is time to consider more constructive options than transmigration as far as the economic development of Indonesia is concerned. In particular it will be argued that in a land scarce country such as Indonesia, but where cheap labour is in abundance, industrial based development is likely to be the most suitable development strategy. Agricultural based transmigration, which involves the search for scarce land and the application of scarce capital would subsequently seem to be especially inopportune. At least it does not justify the effort both inside and outside Indonesia that is currently being put into transmigration, both in absolute terms and relative to the development strategy that is logically implied by Indonesia's factor endowments.

The case for large scale transmigration

Why then has transmigration continued to attract so much interest in Indonesia, and why is it that in various circles aspirations are currently favourable regarding the future role of transmigration? The historical interest in transmigration is related to two major facts about the Indonesian economy. First, Java has never been a rich area of the world, and while it is a very crude and often misleading measure of well being, the average GDP per capita in Java in 1973 was about US $120, while in Malaysia it was US $570, and in Bangladesh it was US $80. About 10 per cent of the Indonesians are estimated to be on a living standard which is consistent with absolute poverty—where an adequate diet cannot be afforded.[3] Most probably the majority of these people are currently living in Java. Like the historic interest in transmigration, the present interest in transmigration is propelled by the 'push' factors of low living standards in Java.

The second major motivation for transmigration has been the 'pull' factor of the other islands. This factor is related to the apparent underpopulation of these islands. Since the Javanese economy is predominantly agricultural, and since so much of the land in the other islands has not been cultivated, it has seemed obvious that the well being of the Javanese may be improved by transmigration in agricultural settlements in

144

the other islands.

Low Javanese productivity and the apparent high land availability on the other islands, have formed the pillars of over 70 years of transmigration policy. The removal of any one of these pillars would immediately eliminate the attractiveness of transmigration. It is curious to note, however, that while in other parts of the world, these two conditions have tended to generate dynamic and unassisted land settlement, in Indonesia land settlement in the last century has been essentially stagnant.

The low level of productivity in Java is unquestionable, as is the familiar picture of the teeming nature of Javanese cultivation high upon the slopes of the mountain sides. It is also unquestionable that the population density in the inner islands of Java, Bali and Madura is many times greater than the most densely populated of the other islands. However, these population densities, expressed in terms of gross land availability, which includes lands that have no economic potential, are obviously not adequate to form a reasonable judgment regarding imbalances in the distribution of the population. A comparison of the population densities in the Sahara Desert and West Germany would not of course indicate that the West Germans should migrate to the Sahara. Clearly what is needed is a measure of population density that takes account of both the economic potential of the population in the numerator and the economic potential of the land in the denominator. In addition it would be desirable to recognise the numerous technological considerations, especially the accumulation of infrastructure, which make certain areas highly productive (this is especially true of industrial and urban areas), despite high population densities. Often the term 'population pressure' is used indiscriminately to cover a multitude of potentially vacuous economic phenomena. The mere presence of large numbers of people in a confined area is clearly not the equivalent of 'population pressure'. Concern is usually only raised when low productivity may lead to poverty. However, this is not necessarily related to the number of people. It is more meaningful to speak of pressure on resources than population pressure per se, if only because the latter terminology often suggests birth control and policies such as population movement, whereas the former lays emphasis more positively on the expansion of the resource base to meet the needs of the people.

No serious attempt is made here to construct an index of population densities that may meaningfully be applied to form judgments on the appropriateness of transmigration. Rather, our objective is the negative one, of showing how difficult it is to form rough and ready judgments about purported imbalances in the distribution of the population. The first column in Table 7.1 expresses the total population as a ratio of the total land area in the various parts of the archipelago. This ratio or variants of it, are frequently being deployed to justify transmigration as a means of rectifying the imbalance in the distribution of the population. The population density is indeed twelve times greater in Java than in Sulawesi, and about 60 times greater than in Kalimantan. The second column in Table 7.1 expresses the ratio of the rural population to the area of land that is regarded as being suitable for agricultural purposes. However crude and unreliable this index may be, it is very much less so than the by now familiar appeals to gross population densities which are often voiced by the proponents of transmigration, regardless of their transparent meaninglessness. This index at least omits some of the population whose livelihoods are most probably not related to the land, as well as including that land that is of supermarginal economic value.

Table 7.1

Population density per sq. km. (1976)

	Gross area a	Net area b
Java, Bali and Madura	637	4,492
Sumatera	51	3,185
Kalimantan	11	c
Sulawesi	51	758
Other	13	2,607
Total	71	3,126

a Total population ÷ total area.
b Rural population ÷ area of land in categories 1-3.
c Kalimantan has no land in categories 1-3.

Instead of Java, Bali, and Madura being 60 times more densely populated than Kalimantan, the net area criterion would if anything suggest the contrary. The differential between Java, Bali and Madura and Sumatera is dramatically reduced by this measure of the net area criterion, indeed to the point where, given the uncertainties inherent in land categorisation and the appropriateness of the numerator, there is probably no significant difference between the two.

Naturally, other ratios could be selected with different numerators and denominators, suggesting greater or smaller imbalances. Unfortunately, up to a point it would be difficult to discriminate between them. A logical case therefore has yet to be made that there is a significantly large imbalance in the geographical distribution of the population that would imply a role for large scale transmigration in the Indonesian archipelago. Most probably, there is no more imbalance in the geographical distribution of the Indonesian population than there is in say France, the US or Egypt. At least one should proceed with this assumption until the contrary is demonstrated to a reasonable degree of satisfaction.

The principles and practice of land settlement

Transmigration in its various forms has been a vehicle of land settlement. Therefore any discussion of transmigration will be incomplete without an assessment of whether or not it serves as a suitable vehicle for land settlement. In particular, what should be the role of the authorities in the land settlement process? This of course is a very large subject, and has been reviewed in Chapter 6. Here we may only discuss the main results.

Nature abhors a vacuum. This basic principle is equally true of the land settlement process. If land is available which affords better prospects than settled land at the margin, the pattern of land settlement will alter in favour of the more productive land. The essence of this marginal productivity theory is that land will on the whole be settled where its marginal product is expected to be the highest. Subsequently, along the frontier of the land that is settled, the marginal productivity of the land will be roughly equal. Differences in productivity might reflect, for example, differences in climate,tastes, transportation linkages, etc.

Virtually the entire history of land settlement throughout the world has been a spontaneous development reflecting the dynamics of the marginal productivity theory, as well as political pressure. On the whole, people have migrated on the basis of improving their economic and social well being. They have seized on land settlement opportunities where they have deemed it to be in their best interest. This was as true in the case of the settlement of North America in the last two centuries, as it was in the times of Abraham, and as it is in many areas of South America today.

If the pattern of land settlement reflects the self-interest of the settlers—what is the legitimate role of government in the land settlement process? In practice, there may be natural constraints to spontaneous and unassisted land settlement which might be easier for the authorities to contend with than the individuals themselves. For example, land beyond the frontier which has good economic potential might not be settled because the private entry costs are prohibitive. The presence of an access road would reduce the settlement costs for the individual, but nobody is prepared to be the first settled. In other words, the social costs of settlement are below the private costs of settlement. The authorities should undertake the construction of access roads since this reduces the divergence between social and private settlement costs in a way that is socially beneficial. The same principle applies to malarial eradication and the like, where what is too expensive for the individual might be quite cheap for society as a whole.

The narrowing of the divergence between social and private settlement costs (as well as the usual roles of government regarding land titling, the maintenance of law and order, etc. etc.) is the basis for the legitimate involvement on the part of the authorities in the land settlement process. This principle does not imply an initiating role on the part of the authorities in the land settlement process; only a secondary but nonetheless important role as a 'trouble-shooter'.

Indeed, the evidence suggests that where the authorities have tried to be initiators in the land settlement process, the results have been particularly unsuccessful:

> ... that few spheres of economic development have a history of, or reputation for, failure to match that of government sponsored colonisation in humid tropical zones. Horror stories abound about expensive ventures that resulted in colonies where few, if any, settlers remained after several years ... The evidence is irrefutable, and failure can be attributed only to the institutions responsible for selecting the areas and the colonists, planning and executing the development programme, and subsequently maintaining or abandoning the infrastructure and services in the region.[4]

Furthermore, there is a conflict between the spirit of pioneering and the prepackaged nature of government directed land settlement.

> Deliberate programmes for settler recruitment have constituted a failure element; self-reliant pioneer colonists are not necessarily attracted by the programmes, and the executive agency tends to be drawn into expensive, paternalistic operations. (Nelson, p.273)

The wrong settlers are chosen, then. Indeed, the only reliable selection process would seem to be that of nature herself.

Care should be taken in interpreting these observations. The crucial test is not whether government directed ventures have failed, but whether there was a significant incidence of failure related to the unassisted ventures on the supermarginal lands. Failure on marginal lands is of course to be expected, and it is possible that the government might be tempted to settle submarginal lands i.e. where the unassisted settler does not wish to go. Nelson suggests that the incidence of failure was indeed significant.

> In all of these cases, as in the directed pioneer projects, viable agriculture proved to be possible. The success or failure of the projects depended on the institutional conditions that guided the proportions of the production factors in the exploitation of the region. The directed projects were saddled with high public expenditures and a rigid design based on information that could not be as accurate as assumed without excessive expenditures for studies on hydrology, sociology, anthropology,

soils, and so on. Spontaneous primary settlement was not burdened by high overheads, and projects launched in the consolidation phase had the benefit of a considerable accumulation
of information on the factors listed above. (p.275)

In other words, government directed settlement projects have tended
to fail for at least three main reasons: (a) the difficulties inherent in
selecting pioneers; (b) the lack of flexibility inherent in organised
settlements; (c) underestimates of risks given the information base.

Dozier[5] too notes that 'adequate and fruitful evidence exists that not
even the most bountiful combination of other conditions can be effective without the proper kind of colonists to go with it' (p.198) and that
it will seem that a 'real danger exists in overproviding and overplanning
for the colonists to the extent that independence and incentive disappear,
will never develop'. (p.206) In other words, there is an inherent conflict
between formal selection procedures which tend to attract dependent
people and the needs of the land beyond the frontier which are for independent and highly motivated pioneers.

There have been several comparative studies of the economic success
of unassisted and directed settlements. Apart from Nelson's results
which indicate that the private and unassisted settler is more likely to
succeed, (p. 264), Dozier notes that '... we find examples of spontaneous
colonists whose returns are considerably higher than those of neighbour-
ing colonists on directed projects in the same tropical forest setting'. (p.
205) Likewise, in the Philippines, Horokova[6] shows that the unassisted
settlers have out-performed the assisted settlers on the basis of a variety
of different economical and social criteria, and Fitzgerald reports for
Kalimantan[7]

Field evidence suggests strongly that the most successful settlers
are those pioneering largely as a result of their own initiative ...
The least successful pioneers would seem to be government
sponsored.

Past experience in various parts of the world emphasises the highly
political nature of land settlement and of the movement of peoples. No
attempt will be made here to discuss the politics of land settlement, only
to observe that there is no endemic reason why land settlement should
inevitably fall under government control and sponsorship. Instead, our
remarks are directed at the economic interest that various vested interests might have in the politics of transmigration.

In the Indonesian case, most probably the high degree of government
control is largely attributable to the direct economic interests that civil
servants have in the bureaucratisation of land settlement in transmigration (as well as other areas too). The profits from corruption inevitably
favour a political economy of extensive government involvement, and

the administration has the power to further its own interests. At the other end of the bureaucracy, the so called beneficiaries of transmigration are politically powerless, since they are dependent on the favours of the civil servants who are after all transferring resources to them from the community at large. Such a system is inherently prone to abuse and the result is usually stagnation rather than economic and social development.

A second important factor behind the high degree of government involvement is the poor quality of the land in the other islands that is available for transmigration. In Latin America and especially Brazil, where there is an abundance of prospective supermarginal land, land settlement does not need to be pushed since through the dynamics of the marginal productivity theory it happens naturally. By contrast, in Indonesia the unsettled land or alternatively the land that is still under shifting cultivation, are submarginal (the reason why they are empty in the first place), given the scarcity of capital, and in accordance with the marginal productivity theory, land settlement and related migration are virtually absent. In this situation the authorities are politically tempted to provide artificial stimuli to land settlement through the provision of subsidies and an inefficient allocation of capital for land settlement where the economic rates of return are unduly low.

The fear is that if the authorities were to pursue a market oriented land settlement policy, there will be little or no transmigration. This would only happen if the land itself did not justify it. If this were the case, the reality would have to be accepted. However, if such basic realities are not accepted, serious economic development can scarcely begin.

These observations at best suggest that the Indonesian authorities alter the design of their transmigration policies in a fundamental fashion since they directly initiate land settlement on a comprehensive basis, and concentrate instead on the less ambitious role of 'trouble shooter' by mainly providing infrastructure in a way that profitably reduces the divergence between private and social settlement costs. At worst they suggest that the authorities should withdraw from transmigration altogether. However, this would only be necessary if the lands beyond the frontier are not attractice enough in themselves to induce unassisted settlement. Unfortunately soil reviews indicate this to be the case. The absence of satisfactory soils makes any discussion of transmigration largely academic.

Indonesia's development strategy

These arguments do not indicate that transmigration in the settlement of new lands can be expected to play an even minor role in the economic and social development of Indonesia. However, it is often asked, if the other islands do not have the economic potential to permit a reasonably ambitious programme of transmigration, what other options do the Indonesians have in averting the ever threatening overpopulation of Java? If indeed transmigration is recommended on these grounds, this paper would suggest that Indonesia's prospects are dire indeed. Even if as has already been argued, the threat of overpopulation in Java has been overplayed, before transmigration may be demoted as an integral part of Indonesia's development strategy, it is necessary to identify development options more constructive than transmigration.

Clearly a blueprint for Indonesian economic development cannot be included here, yet a number of striking pointers exist. Despite the advent of the Green Revolution, the agricultural sector which in Indonesia accounts for about 44 per cent of GDP and 68 per cent of the labour force, has only grown by about 4 per cent per year, whereas the overall growth rate of GDP has been in excess of 7 per cent per year. Moreover, as marginal lands come under cultivation agricultural growth has every prospect of decelerating. Despite the vast open spaces on the other islands, it has been increasingly recognised that Indonesia is a land scarce community. It is also a capital scarce community. Its main resource is its labour force which is essentially hard working and shows every indication of adaptability to changed economic stimuli.[8]

Many other Southeast Asian countries have found themselves in a similar situation to Indonesia—of land and capital scarcity, where cheap labour is in abundance. Hong Kong, Korea, Taiwan, Japan and others at various times and under stimuli not significantly different to those prevailing in Indonesia, have embarked upon an industrial development strategy, using the reserves of cheap labour to add value in the process of light manufacturing at first and then heavy manufacturing at maturity. It must seriously be asked why, despite the same kind of impulses, Indonesia has failed to follow what might loosely be called the Southeast Asian model of industrial development. Indeed, this is most probably the greatest puzzle about the Indonesian economy.

Some believe that Indonesia is not an exception, and is on the verge of taking off. Indeed one study (under preparation by Prof. A. Strout of MIT) envisages that it is only a matter of time before Indonesia follows some of her neighbours down the path of development through industrialisation. Indeed the world economic consequences of such a development on the part of a nation of 130 million could be major and a possible obstacle for the Indonesians to overcome.

A number of obvious constraints to growth, however, may be identified, some of which are more easy to remedy than others. The expropriations during the Sukarno era have done much to dampen private initiative both domestically and internationally as far as the Indonesian economy is concerned, and only time and appropriate government policies will restore a more favourable climate for private initiative. In addition, the widespread practice of corruption acts as a tax on entrepreneurial initiative which is bound to put Indonesian businessmen at a disadvantage over their overseas competitors both regarding domestic and overseas markets. The comparative advantage of cheap labour can easily be spoiled by a comparative disadvantage generated by bribery and corruption. While the eradication of corruption can only be hoped for, fiscal measures may be explored to offset the explicit taxes on initiative that corruption generates.[9]

Another major constraint may be identified as the exchange rate which is most probably seriously overvalued. Since the devaluation against the dollar in 1971, Indonesian price levels have risen by about 50 per cent in relation to world price levels expressed in dollars. An overvalued exchange rate will have a deindustrialising influence on the economy, since it stifles the development of import substitution at the same time as reducing the profitability of exporting. This overvaluation has become particularly serious since the oil price hikes of 1973-74, and the climate is being established that will not only hinder future economic development, but which will also undermine existing achievements in the development of the industrial and agricultural sectors alike.

It would also seem that there is considerable scope for improving labour policy, which at present mitigates in favour of capital which is scarce rather than labour which is in abundance. Thus, what growth Indonesia achieves is to some extent malignant rather than balanced. Alternatively, a more efficient growth path may be achieved if the restrictions on labour imposed by present labour market policies are relaxed.

Infrastructure is a further prerequisite to industrial growth. In many parts of Indonesia roads are impassable in the rainy season, power supplies are unreliable, telecommunications are poor. While the provision of satisfactory infrastructure cannot, of course, guarantee development, its absence can obviously impede it when the other circumstances appear conducive to development. For example, farmgate prices are inordinately below market prices simply because of the difficulties in transporting the outputs no more than fifty miles to the market place. In an international setting, the absence of satisfactory infrastructure is bound to place Indonesia at a serious disadvantage.

These remarks are not of course intended to form the basis of a development strategy for Indonesia, although it does appear that there is much that may be done at the macroeconomic level to improve matters. A task force on the causes of Indonesia's economic backwardness in the context of the development of her Southeast Asian neighbours could form the basis of a development strategy for Indonesia.

Conclusions

These remarks, while inimical to transmigration, are intended to be constructive in the sense that the talents and efforts that are being invested into transmigration policy would most probably bear more fruits in other areas regarding the Indonesian economy. At the very least these efforts are disproportionate to any contributions transmigration is likely to make to the Indonesians. The search for suitable transmigration projects seems to be reminiscent of the search for the needle in the haystack. The debate of whether or not the needle exists is in danger of making the entire issue both boring and ridiculous. The time has surely come to move on to more fruitful pastures.

Notes

1   B. White, 'Population, involution and employment in Rural Java', *Development and Change,* Vol. 7, 1976, p.268.
2   In a study being prepared by Dr W. S. Johnson, of Ball State University, Indiana.
3   Based on the discussion in Chapter 5.
4   M. Nelson, *The Development of Tropical Lands; Policies Used in Latin America,* The Johns Hopkins University Press, Baltimore and London, 1973, p.265.
5   Craig L. Dozier, *Land Development Colonisation in Latin America,* Frederick A. Praeger, New York, 1969.
6   Eva Horokova, *Problems of Filipino Settlers,* Occasional Paper No.4, Institute of Southeast Asian Studies, Singapore.
7   Dennis P. Fitzgerald, 'Pioneer Settlement in Southern and East Kalimantan'.
8   See J. B. Donges, B. Stecher, and F. Wolter, *Industrial Development Policies for Indonesia,* J. C. Mohr (Paul Siebeck), Tubingen, 1974, pp.40-44.
9   See M. Beenstock, 'Corruption and Development', *World Development,* January 1979.

8   The economics of shifting cultivation

Introduction

Shifting cultivation may be regarded as the most extensive of agricultural systems in terms of factor usages on the spectrum of agricultural techniques. At the most sophisticated end of this spectrum the agricultural system tends to be highly capital intensive in terms of machinery, the use of fertilizers and high yielding varieties etc. Shifting cultivation which is marked by the virtual absence of all forms of capital occupies the position at the opposite end of this imaginary spectrum. However, in its own way shifting cultivation is as rational and as sophisticated as modern agricultural technology and may be regarded in the first instance as a rational response to economic and social forces expressed in terms of relative factor availabilities, the state of agricultural technology and the cultural constraints and aspirations of the shifting cultivators themselves. By the same token, the evolution from shifting cultivation to permanent cultivation along the routes of semipermanent systems and ley farming may be understood in terms of the changing balance between these social and economic forces.[1]

Primeval agriculture has been based on shifting cultivation as much because of the high availability of land as because of the absence of a technology to support a permanent cultivation. In this section the interplay of forces between factor availabilities and the balance between permanent and shifting cultivation are explored. The obvious justification for this analysis is that a considerable proportion of agricultural land is still under shifting cultivation although this proportion is falling. In addition, where capital is scarce shifting cultivation is more likely to emerge as the most efficient farming technique, relying as it were on nature's own capital rather than man made capital. Thus the planter who is considering the establishment of permanent settlements in areas which are currently under shifting cultivation should stop to consider whether or not he is misallocating scarce resources. It may be the case that in certain areas shifting cultivation is in fact a rational land use.

In Java shifting cultivation has virtually disappeared in response to population pressures. In Sumatra the same tendency is happening. However, as much as about 46 per cent of agricultural land in the provinces of Lampung, South Sumatra and Bengkulu was under shifting cultivation in 1972.[2] Since at any one time shifting cultivators only farm about 10 per cent of the land, the proportion of land currently engaged in shifting cultivation is much smaller than this. However, the relevant statistic for the land under shifting cultivation is the fallow plus the cropped land.

Basic principles

As a stable system of agriculture shifting cultivation relies on a sequence of cropping and fallow periods which is compatible with the avoidance of alang-alang (in Indonesia) as a climax vegetation. Alang-alang only becomes a climax vegetation when the fertility of the soil under shifting cultivation has fallen below a critical level, or when repeated burnings have eradicated the stock of forest seedlings in the soil.[3] Below this level of soil fertility the more aggressive alang-alang dominates the recovery of the secondary forest and what was originally primary or secondary forest is eventually transformed into man made grasslands. Above this level of fertility the opposite happens and the forest eventually recovers to dominate the alang-alang. A viable system of shifting cultivation therefore requires that the fertility of the soil should not be depleted below this critical level.

If an alang-alang climax vegetation is induced, the fertility of the soil remains fairly stable. Alang-alang does not harm the soil; it merely prevents it from improving to a level that is once again suitable for cultivation. As it were, alang-alang areas go out of circulation from the merry-go-round of shifting cultivation.

In Figure 8.1, this critical level of fertility is indicated by Ox. However, the farmer may maintain land within circulation by using a variety of techniques. For example if he crops the land for a short period of time (one year) the fertility of the land will inevitably recover faster than if the land is cropped for a longer period. Let us assume that the initial fertility of the soil is 0a. The initial burn will raise the fertility to b and one year's cropping will reduce it to c. If the farmer then rests the land for say nine years the fertility is restored to g and the farmer may repeat the cycle i.e., ghij—a ten-year stable system of cultivation. On the other hand, if instead he crops the land for a second consecutive year the fertility will fall to d. On the diagram cd is drawn greater than bc to denote the possibility that the rate of fertility depletion increases with cropping. However, the precise pattern will vary from case to case. Since the fertility of d is greater than x the land does not go out of cultivation. Instead, the fertility gradually recovers so that at k the original fertility is restored. The precise recovery rate will once again vary from case to case. However, most probably the recovery rate represented by the slope of dk and cg will eventually vary inversely with the

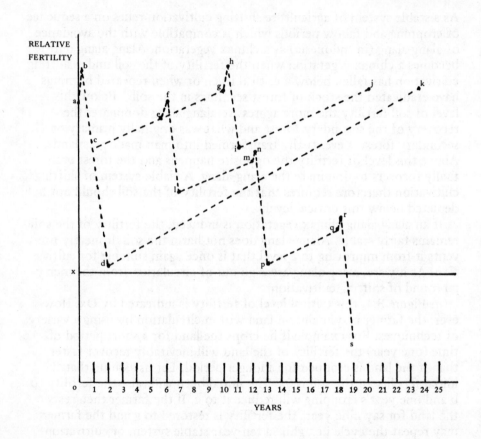

Figure 8.1 Soil fertility patterns under shifting cultivation

156

loss of fertility through cropping.

Both these cropping patterns are stable. Let us assume however, that in the case of the first cropping pattern the farmer crops the land during the seventh year instead of waiting until the eleventh year when fertility has completely recovered. The burn in this case will inevitably be weaker (fe is smaller than ba) since there will be less to burn and after one year's cropping fertility falls to 1. If this cycle is repeated then during the fourth round the fertility of the soil falls below x and goes out of circulation. This cycle is an unstable system of shifting cultivation.

The optimal cycle

Out of the set of stable systems of shifting cultivation some will be more efficient than others and at least one will be the most efficient. In the previous example the cycle abghij is more efficient than the cycle abcdk for two reasons. First, the former cycle is shorter since there are only nine years of fallow per cropping year to the latter's eleven years. This is due to the slower recovery rate of the second system. Secondly, the yield of the second cropping year in the latter case will be lower than the yield in the first case because the fertility in the second year is lower. On the other hand the relevant comparison is the present value of the crop in which case the second system has an obvious advantage over the first in that the second crop is brought in nine years ahead of the second crop in the first system. But the third crop of the first system arrives five years ahead of the third crop of the second system.

The optimal system will maximize the present value of the crop over a given time horizon. For illustrative purposes three stable systems are analysed:

Table 8.1

Patterns of shifting cultivation

Case	Yield profile	Fallow years	Present value
A	100	9	233.4
B	100 90	20	258.0
C	100 90 40	39	238.6

In the case A the land is cropped for 1 year at a time and left fallow for 9 years. The yield is always 100. In case B the land is cropped for 2 years at a time and then left fallow for 20 years. The yield in the second year is assumed to drop to 90 and there are 10 fallow years for every cropping year. In case C there is a sharp drop in the yield for the

157

for the third consecutive cropping year and there are 13 fallow years for every cropping year. Using a 5 per cent annual discount rate the present values of the various systems are compared (computed over a period of 51 years). Case B emerges as the optimal system of shifting cultivation since the deterioration in the cropping yeild and the fallow/cropping ratio is not sufficient to out balance the value of the earlier cropping than case A. Cases A and C are roughly comparable systems of shifting cultivation in terms of their respective present values. As the discount rate is increased case C would become increasingly attractive and beyond a point case B would lose out to case C as the optimum system.

In practice the optimum will depend on the details of yield profiles, fertility recovery rates and the time preferences of the shifting cultivators themselves.

Comparative agriculture

So far we have assumed that the only agricultural choice was the length of the cycle of shifting cultivation and that there was only one form of agricultural output. In the absence of capital the farmer is most probably forced into shifting cultivation for annual food production since he has to rely on nature to restore fertility to the land. Under these circumstances the economic problem that confronts him is how to allocate his time between shifting cultivation for food and the production of perennials which necessarily must be the basis of permanent agriculture. The optimal allocation will occur when his marginal product is equated between these two competing activities.

When capital is available the farmer has the option of producing food on the basis of semipermanent or permanent cultivation since he may buy fertilizer to assist the natural recovery of the land's fertility. In the limit he may replace the natural processes entirely, in which event the land comes under permanent cultivation. Investment in fertilizers would tend in any event to speed up the cycle of shifting cultivation since the fertility recovery rate is accelerated. In addition, of course, the underlying fertility of the soil may be enhanced.

The microeconomic issues that are involved in evaluating the relative merits of shifting and permanent cultivation as far as fertilizer use is concerned may once more be illustrated by comparing present values. We consider a piece of land that may be farmed once every ten years under shifting cultivation or every year under permanent cultivation. The only difference between the two cases is that in the second case the fertility lost is replenished with fertilizer. However, a disadvantage of permanent cultivation is the extra weeding and land tilling costs that

are avoided under shifting cultivation. A farmer would be indifferent
between permanent and shifting cultivation when:

$$\sum_{i=1}^{\infty} \left(\frac{Y - X}{1+r}\right)^i = \frac{Y}{1+r} + \sum_{i=1}^{\infty} \left(\frac{Y}{1+r}\right)^{hi}$$

i.e. when the present value of the benefits of farming land under permanent cultivation is equal to the present value of the benefits under
shifting cultivation, where:

Y = yield per year
r = discount rate
X = annual weeding plus fertilizer costs etc.
h = length of cropping cycle in years plus one

Taking case A of the previous section as our example of shifting
cultivation Y is 100 and h is eleven. If we apply a discount rate of 5 per
cent the solution for X is 88.33. Thus if the costs of fertilizer etc. are
below 88.33 it is better to use the land for permanent cultivation and
vice versa.

In practice the problem is not so dichotomous since there is an infinite spectrum between the two poles of permanent and shifting cultivation. The intensity of land rotation will vary inversely with the cost of
fertilizer and the availability of capital for its purchase. Alternatively,
technical progress is likely to generate a shift along this spectrum in
favour of permanent cultivation since it effectively reduces investment
costs (X) and increases the productivity of capital. Following this
analogy, therefore, technical progress in agriculture is likely to enhance
capital intensive agriculture and reduce the importance of shifting
cultivation. At any point in time, however, both forms of agriculture
will be observed since the comparative advantage of certain areas might
still lie with shifting cultivation, i.e. the capital investments in these
lands would be too high to warrant their inclusion under permanent
cultivation. Agricultural dualism of this nature subsequently has an
obvious economic interpretation.

Agricultural dynamics

The formula derived in the previous section sheds light on the dynamics
that are involved in the evolution between shifting and permanent

cultivation. The formula is more conveniently expressed as:*

$$\frac{(Y - X)}{r} = \frac{Y}{(1 + r)^{h-1}-1}$$

It may be shown (by the binomial expansion) that

$$(1 + r)^{h-1} -1 > r$$

in which case the present value of the benefits of permanent cultivation are more sensitive to Y than its counterpart under shifting cultivation. In the absence of population pressures and related pressures on the land the value of the crop yield (Y) will be constant over time. If land is in abundance the supply curve of food will be infinitely elastic; where each additional person becomes a shifting cultivator in the seemingly endless forest. However, when the point is reached at which there is not enough land to go around the price of food will begin to rise reflecting the scarcity of the land and Y will begin to rise. The present value of the benefits of both shifting and permanent agriculture will rise; however, the latter will rise proportionately faster than the former as is demonstrated by the formula, in which case permanent cultivation will become attractice relative to shifting cultivation and the entire spectrum of agricultural production will shift its emphasis in the direction of permanent cultivation away from shifting cultivation.

It is in this way that population pressure eventually reduces and even eliminates shifting agriculture in favour of permanent agriculture. The dynamic factors are in effect twofold with shifting cultivation getting caught as it were between the closing scissors of population growth on the one hand and technical progress on the other, both of which in the light of the present analysis would lead to a decline in the relative importance of shifting agriculture.

Policy considerations

It is sometimes argued that shifting cultivation is inefficient and that land which is currently under shifting cultivation should be rehabilitated and put into permanent cultivation. Often these arguments reflect a bourgeois political attitude in which at best the nomad or the itinerant have no place or at worst are a source of political embarrassment for those that are concerned with the cosmetics of economic development.

* i.e. observing e.g. that:
  $$a + a^3 + a^6 = (1-a^{6 + 3})/1-a^3$$

160

On the whole, however, nature tends to look after herself in a reasonably efficient fashion and the transition between different methods of cultivation is likely to take place in a relatively painless way if these natural processes are not forced or artificially impeded. Society on the whole tends to adapt its agricultural techniques in a rational way to the economic and social forces that prevail. In particular if capital is scarce and the land low yielding shifting agriculture could persist despite apparent population pressure. Alternatively, discrimination against shifting cultivation would lead to an unnecessary profitless misallocation of resources.

Notes

1   As argued by E. Boserup, *The Conditions of Agricultural Growth*, Allen and Unwin, London, 1965.
2   See *South Sumatera Regional Planning Study*, Land Use Reports (University of Bonn).
3   A number of useful references may be consulted. See in particular *The Soil Under Shifting Cultivation*, by P. H. Nye and D. J. Greenland, Commonwealth Agricultural Bureau 1961, England. This publication is particularly useful on the technical and agronomic aspects of shifting cultivation. A less technical presentation is in H. Ruthenberg, *Farming Systems in the Tropics*, Clarendon Press, Oxford England, 1971. See also K. J. Pelzer, *Pioneer Settlement in the Asiatic Tropics*, American Geographical Society, 1945, Chapter 2. For cultural and related aspects of shifting cultivation see J. E. Spencer, *Shifting Cultivation in Southeast Asia*, University of California Publications in Geography, Vol. 19, 1966.

9 Urban development and the determinants of migration

Introduction

The model of rural-urban migration suggested by Todaro (1969) has been regarded as an important intellectual framework for analysing migration and urban unemployment in developing countries. Important features of this model are the assumption that the urban wage is fixed at some relatively high level and that the volume of urban unemployment will serve as an adjustment mechanism in dualistic labour markets under the assumption that the flow of migration will depend on the level of the expected urban-rural income differential.

The so called Harris-Todaro Model (HTM) has since been modified and developed in a number of useful respects (e.g. Collier (1975), Fields (1975)). However, the comments in this chapter focus almost exclusively on the basic version of HTM that was unveiled in Harris-Todaro (1970). In particular our concern is with the specification of the rural-urban migration schedule in HTM which has largely been carried over in the various subsequent developments on the basic model. This specification relates the flow of migration to the level of the expected wage differential[1] which implies that in equilibrium the expected urban wage will equal the rural wage.

The difficulty with this specification is that it ignores risk when in fact it would seem that risk is an integral feature of HTM. For example, Harris and Todaro (1970, p.127) depict the finding of urban employment in terms of a 'periodic random job selection process ... whenever the number of available jobs is exceeded by the number of job seekers'. Thus in every period the urban migrant stands an equal chance of being one of the lucky ones to be picked for a job. Even if we assume that he is certain about his chances (as in HTM) the expected urban wage will be a random variable and the prospective migrant will have to take into consideration the riskiness of the expected urban income as well as the expected rural income itself. If he does this, the aggregate migration schedule will not be generally of the form in HTM and the expected urban wage will not necessarily equal the rural wage in equilibrium. Instead, the flow of migration will depend on the change rather than the level of the expected income differential and in equilibrium there will generally be a differential or risk premium between the expected urban wage and rural wage. Also this specification may alter the

162

relationship HTM postulated between urban job creation and migration under urban minimum wage regulations. These propositions are developed in the next sections.

Various wider aspects of HTM[2] are not considered here. For example, multiple period optimisation is not taken into consideration, nor are the implications of the various search models, migration costs, the role of the informal sector etc., etc. Our ground rules are precisely those that appear in Harris and Todaro (1970) which serve as a useful enough basis for introducing a discussion of risk in a fairly comprehensive way.

Risk and risk aversion

Unfortunately HTM does not discuss the nature of the agricultural wage in any detail. Thus whereas the expected urban wage is acknowledged as a risky random variable the status of the agricultural or rural wage is unclear as far as risk is concerned. In practice, as most farmers will testify, the agricultural wage is risky too depending inter alia on the vagaries of the weather, diseases and pests and the vicissitudes of agricultural prices. Therefore, in what follows we assume that the agricultural wage (W_a) is risky, but that it is less risky than the expected urban wage (W_a^e), and that the expected urban wage happens to be greater than the agricultural wage (otherwise we have no story). On Figure 9.1 therefore, the co-ordinates regarding expected wage rates and risk for the rural sector are at X and those for the urban sector are initially Y_1.

We begin by considering the decision criteria of the individual prospective migrant and assume that he seeks to maximise his expected utility. His expected utility function is of the familiar form in that expected utility is a positive function of the expected wage and a negative function or risk, i.e., he is risk averse. Such a utility function would be represented by a set of indifference curves on the diagram which were convex to the horizontal axis and where expected utility rose as the co-ordinates moved in a north or westerly direction. This criterion function is appropriate in the context of rural-urban migration as conceived in HTM because it takes account of both the risk and the expected return on migration which is explicit in the situation proposed by Harris and Todaro.

Although it is not essential to the argument, we assume that the individual has to live in the urban sector or the rural sector; he cannot work in two places during the same period. Subsequently, he must choose between X and Y_1.[3] This implies that if he maximises his expected utility a corner solution will obtain; either he will be happiest in the urban sector or the rural sector. A number of possibilities are discussed in relation to Figure 9.1. Consider the preference maps for individual A (of which AX is a member) and individual B (of which BY_1 is a member). Given the shape of his preference function and his relative aversion to risk A will be at a corner solution at X since in his calculus Y_1 is inferior. On the other hand, the opposite holds for B who maximises expected utility at Y_1. Consequently A will choose to live in the rural sector and B in the urban sector.

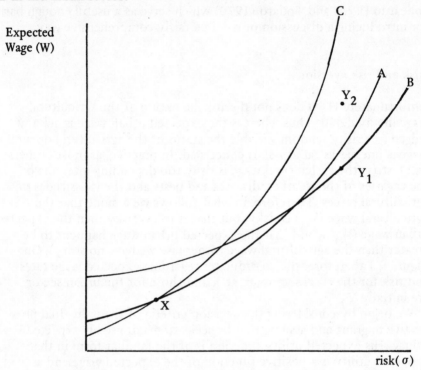

Figure 9.1 Rural-urban migration decision

Consider next what happens when the expected urban wage rises but everything else remains unchanged. The risk expected wage co-ordinates in the urban sector rise vertically to Y_2. B will of course remain in the urban sector since urban employment is now even more attractive to him. But A will shift his corner solution from X to Y_2 since given his preference map X will be inferior to Y_2; the increase in the expected urban wage has more than compensated for the additional risk. Subsequently A will migrate to the urban sector.

However, C will still prefer to stay in the rural sector. But as the expected urban wage rises (ceteris paribus) a point will be reached when even C will feel that the expected benefits of migrating dominates his high assessment of risk. The converse would happen if the expected rural-urban wage differential were to fall; a point could be reached where even B opted to migrate from the urban sector to the rural sector.

If this decision logic is applied on an economy-wide basis, it implies that the proportion of the population that will desire to live in the urban sector will depend on the difference between the level of the expected urban-rural wage differential (for given risk relativities), and that the flow of migration which is based on the change in this proportion will subsequently depend on the change in the expected wage differential and not its level as has been assumed in HTM. By the same token, the proportion of the population that will desire to live in the urban sector will depend on the level of the risk differential (for given expected wage differentials), and the flow of migration will subsequently depend on the change in this risk differential.

Therefore, whereas in HTM the migration schedule is of the form

$$M = F \ (W_u^e - W_a) \tag{9.1}$$

where M is the flow of rural-urban migration,[4] the foregoing analysis implies that the basic form of the function should be

$$M = H \ (\dot{W}_u^e - \dot{W}_a, \ \dot{\sigma}_u - \dot{\sigma}_a) \tag{9.2}$$

where σ_u and σ_a are the risk factors in the respective sectors H_1 will be positive and H_2 will be negative. While recognising the obvious importance of risk in equation (9.2), in what follows we assume that σ_u and σ_a are constant since this was the assumption implicit in HTM.

If however, $\sigma_u = \sigma_a$, i.e., both wages are equally risky, then under the circumstances depicted on Figure 9.1, Y_1 would be vertically above X, in which case all the corner solutions would occur at Y_1. Under these circumstances all the population would seek to live in the urban sector and the expected urban wage would be driven into line with the rural wage as Harris and Todaro argue. Alternatively, if everybody were unaverse to risk, i.e., if all the indifference curves were horizontal lines, the same would happen; everybody would wish to live in the urban sector. Under either of these circumstances H_1 would be infinite (or as large as the population itself). In practice the resulting flow of migration might not be instantaneous on account of lags due to organisational delays etc., and in econometric estimation it would be desirable to specify a distributed lag. A version of such a lag is that the flow of migration is related to the level of the wage differential, i.e., the long run of infinity is approached at a uniform rate over time.

In terms of the analysis that has been presented, this would be the interpretation of the migration schedule in HTM. Needless to say, it can hardly be considered as being sufficiently general either on theoretical grounds, or even as an econometric strategy that may be used under what amount to an extreme set of assumptions.

Risk and equilibrium

Without intending to become involved in the welfare indexation problem
it is helpful to conceive of the set of community indifference curves
when considering the expected urban-rural differential in equilibrium.
These curves will be of the same form as their individual counterparts
in Figure 9.1 and a representative curve is shown on Figure 9.2. As
before we assume that the urban wage is riskier than the rural wage in
which case

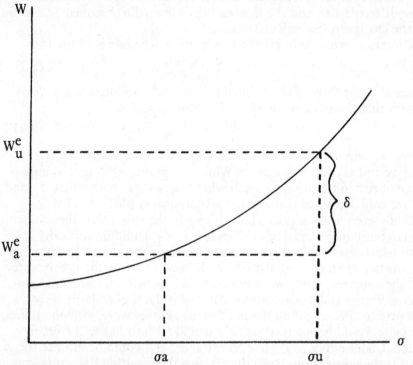

Figure 9.2 Risk and equilibrium

$\sigma_u > \sigma_a$. The expected rural wage is assumed to be W_a^e.

Equilibrium will prevail when the flow of migration has stopped, or
in terms of our analysis where society as a whole is indifferent between
the rural and urban sectors. In view of the relative risks, this point of
indifference is reached when the expected urban income is W_u^e. In other
words a risk premium of δ is reflected in the expected urban wage and
it will only be when $\delta = 0$ that the result in HTM regarding the equation

166

of W_u^e and W_a^e will obtain. Once again, this would only occur if $\sigma_a = \sigma_u$ or if the indifference curve were horizontal implying zero aversion to risk.

In general δ is likely to be positive in which case W_u^e would tend to be greater than W_a^e in equilibrium. Indeed a number of reported empirical measures of this differential seem to imply that δ is quite large. It may be inferred from Figure 9.2 that δ/W_a^e varies inversely with W_a^e itself as we move successively onto higher indifference curves the marginal social rate of substitution between risk and expected return tends to rise. If this is so, the risk premium measured as a percentage of the real wage is likely to fall with the agricultural wage rate.

Urban job creation and employment

Harris and Todaro (1970, p.132) 'claimed that more than one agricultural worker will likely migrate in response to the creation of one additional industrial job'. Their equilibrium condition is for the expected urban wage to equal the agricultural wage.

$$\overline{W}_m \frac{N_m}{N_u} = W_a \tag{9.3}$$

where

$\overline{W}_m$	is the minimum urban wage
N_m	is the value of urban employment
N_u	is the size of the urban labour force
W_a	is the agricultural wage

It is assumed that $\overline{W}_m > W_a$ and that $N_m < N_u$. Equation (9.3) implies that if an extra job is provided i.e., $\Delta N_m = 1$ more than one worker will migrate to the urban sector since the relationship between N_u and N_m is W_m/W_a which is greater than unity. If relative prices were endogenised and marginal products were assumed to alter this relationship would be modified, but this observation is the nub of the claim in HTM that urban job creation might be destabilising in the presence of an urban minimum wage. Assuming these parameters to be fixed, equation (9.3) suggests the HTM result is not merely likely but inevitable given their specification of the migration schedule.

The alternative specification of the migration schedule that has been suggested here implies a different equilibrium relationship as has been pointed out in the previous section. Because the expected urban wage is assumed to be risky in equilibrium the expected urban wage must be greater than the agricultural wage.

$$\frac{\overline{W}_m N_m}{N_u} = KW_a \qquad K > 1 \qquad (9.4)$$

in which case the relationship between the urban labour force and employment will be

$$N_u = \frac{\overline{W}_m N_m}{K \ W_a}$$

If $K \ W_a > W_m$ the HTM view about the destabilising effects of urban job creation will no longer hold since for every job created less than one person will migrate from the rural sector to the urban sector. Since $K > 1$ it will always be true that the HTM argument will be at the very least muted.[5] The more risk averse prospective migrants are and the riskier the urban wage the greater will be the value of K. In the limit, as K approaches infinity there would be no relationship at all between urban employment and rural-urban migration. Therefore changing the specification of the rural-urban migration schedule in a way that reflects risk may also alter the normative implications of HTM.

Notes

1   Harris and Todaro (1970, p.129).
2   As defined by Harris and Todaro (1970).
3   If he were not so restricted, he could diversify his employment between the two sectors. If there is no covariance between the two wage rates the locum of opportunities would be the line XY_1. If this covariance is negative, the locum becomes convex to the vertical axis and if it is positive the converse happens.
4   Throughout this discussion it is assumed that there is no natural increase in the population.
5   Indeed, previous researchers have noted e.g. Fields (1975) that HTM over-predicts the volume of urban unemployment as would tend to be the case if K is assumed to be unity.

References

Collier, P., 1975, Labour Mobility and Labour Utilization in Developing Countries, *Oxford Bulletin of Economics and Statistics*, 37, August, 169-189.

Fields, G. S., 1975, Rural-Urban Migration, Urban Unemployment and Underemployment, and Job-Search Activity in LDCs, *Journal of Development Economics*, 2, June, 165-187.

Harris, J., and Todaro, M. P., 1970, Migration, Unemployment and Development: a Two Sector Analysis, *American Economic Review*, 60, March, 126-142.

Todaro, M. P., 1969, A Model of Labour Migration and Urban Unemployment in Less Developed Countries, *American Economic Review*, 59, March, 138-48.

10   Some welfare aspects of migrant-employment

Especially among the developing nations the migrant worker has emerged as a significant economic factor.[1] For example at the international level, there are substantial numbers of Tunisians and Algerians working in France, Turks and Yugoslavs in West Germany, Voltaics in Ivory Coast, Pakistanis in Great Britain, Mexicans in the U.S., etc. Also, within developing countries there is an extensive incidence of rural labourers working in the urban areas so that the migrant worker is both a national as well as an international phenomenon.

The objective in this chapter is to introduce a discussion on the welfare implications of migrant working for the host and source regions (or countries). In particular, we focus on the design of what might be an optimal policy on the part of the source region, where the objective is to maximise the economic welfare of the remaining population in the region.[2] Berry and Soligo (1969, pp.781-2) have pointed out[3] that the static effect of emigration in a neoclassical model of production is to reduce the welfare of the population in the source region since '... the intramarginal emigrants had individually contributed more to total product than the marginal unit, but all emigrants were receiving a wage equal to the contribution of the marginal worker'. However, the point at issue here is that migrant workers invariably remit a proportion of their income to the source region in which event the source region also enjoys a direct benefit from its migrant workers as well as the loss previously referred to.

The analysis extends more generally to permanent emigrants who happen to remit part of their incomes rather than just to migrant workers who tend to work on a temporary, if sometimes prolonged basis in the host region. The model, therefore, may offer a richer framework for analysing emigration, 'brain drain', etc., where as a limiting case, the remittance factor is zero. However, emigration is likely to involve the transfer of capital as well as labour and it is for this reason that we focus on the migrant worker who is unlikely to transfer his capital; although only having to consider the transfer of labour raises sufficient complications in its own right.

Welfare analysis

On Figure 10.1 the labour force in the source region (S) is initially Oc while in the host region (H) it is Ok.[4] In this essentially static analysis the respective capital stocks are assumed to be constant while labour in both regions is assumed to be homogenous. The production functions may differ and this is reflected in the nature of the ab and hf schedules. Migrant workers in H are assumed to remit a proportion of their income gh/ch.

In the initial situation GDP in S is represented by the area Oadc and the wage rate which is assumed to be equal to the marginal labour product is Oe. In H, GDP is initially Ohpk and the wage rate is oi. However, jk of the labour force in H are migrant workers from S.[5] Their total earnings are jnpk of which they remit mnpl, therefore GNP in H is represented by Ohpk−mnpl, while GNP is S is Oade + mnpl.

This calculus suggests three distinct welfare aggregates:

(i) GNP_S—the population in the source region whose total income receipts are equal to the GNP of the region.

(ii) GNP_H^*—the indigenous population in the host region (i.e., based on the labour force oj which excludes the migrant workers from the welfare calculus) whose total income receipts are:[6]

$$GNP_H^* = GNP_H - jmlk = Ohpnj$$

In other words, this welfare aggregate is parochial in the sense that the natives of H do not regard migrant workers as part of their own community. Likewise, the first aggregate excludes the migrant workers from the calculus. Thus, the migrant workers are assumed to be a separate community which is alienated from the natives of H as well as their erstwhile compatriots in the source region. This assumption is likely to be more appropriate when H and S are separate countries than when they are separate regions in the source country.

(iii) Y_M—the net income of the migrant workers themselves which is equal to jmlk.

The discussion which follows abstracts from possible terms of trade changes between H and S since in general there is little that may be deduced about them in the absence of empirical estimates.[7] Although the terms of trade are assumed to be unaltered by changes in the members of migrant workers we note that they might affect the welfare calculus in practice. Also, in the event that H and S belong to different currency areas we assume no divergence between shadow and actual exchange rates in which case the fact that remittances are in terms of foreign exchange is of no normative significance. It is further assumed that the migrant worker phenomenon is a one way process.

171

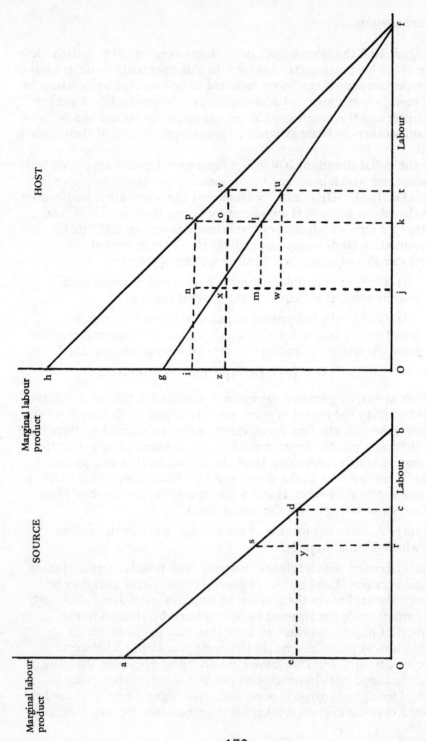

Figure 10.1 Analysis of migrant employment

172

In other words, Turks choose to work in West Germany but West Germans do not choose to work in Turkey. Within developing countries, migrant workers tend to be of rural origin working in the urban areas rather than the other way around. Therefore, the simplifying (but inessential) assumption that H and S may be clearly distinguished is realistic enough.[8]

We now consider the welfare implications when the number of migrant workers rises by $kt = er$ on Figure 10.1. In the source region, GDP falls by rsde but ryde of this represents the income that is foregone by the additional migrant workers. Therefore, under the assumption that these workers did not own any of the capital in S these considerations would imply that the income of the remaining population in S would fall by ysd. In other words, while emigration raises the marginal labour product by ys, average per capita income falls.[9]

In the host region the marginal labour product falls to tu and migrant workers will remit wxvu while retaining jwut. GDP in the host region rises by kpvt but the parochial welfare of H will only increase by xnpv. It is emphasised that this calculus has all the shortcomings of the conventional national income accounting framework since it fails to reflect the utility the migrant workers enjoy from remitting, the disutility associated with family separation, changes in the distribution of income, etc. We may now summarise the net changes in welfare of the three aggregates previously defined.

(i) The change in the welfare of the remaining population in S must reflect the loss of surplus and from the workers who are now working in H as well as the net change in remittances.

$$\Delta \text{GNP}_S^* = \text{ysd} + \text{wxvu} - \text{mnpl}.[10]$$

ΔGNP_S^* may be positive or negative in which case the remaining population in S may or may not be worse off as a consequence of the additional migrant workers. Part of the problem is that there is a 'terms of trade loss' since the previous migrant workers (jk) now earn less and so remit less.

(ii) The change in the welfare of the native population in H is unambiguously positive since

$$\Delta \text{GNP}_H^* = \text{xnpv}$$

However, this improvement involves a redistribution partly at the expense of the native workers (zinx), partly at the expense of the original migrant workers (xnpo) and a surplus on the larger work force (opv). The redistributive effects away from the native work force make migrant employment as politically controversial as it is, especially when H and S are separate countries. Meanwhile, in the host region, the principal

173

beneficiaries are likely to be workers since not only do their wages rise but also they are most probably the recipients of the remittances.

(iii) The original migrant workers are worse off because their net earnings are jw instead of jm. The additional migrant workers are assumed to be better off otherwise they would have preferred to remain at home, i.e. tu > rs. Indeed, migrant workers (and migrants in general) will tend to act as an equilibrating mechanism. If we assume that the criterion for labour allocation is its marginal product, migrant workers will continue to flow from S to H until marginal labour products are equated, or until the differential reflects the net disutility from migrant employment.

Considerations of optimality

The previous discussion raises the policy issue of whether this equilibrium is socially desirable from the point of view of the remaining population in S since in the aggregate they may be better off if they restrict the numbers of migrant workers in H. We thus have the possibility of an 'optimal tariff' situation. However, it is most probably more realistic to conceive of this issue when H and S are separate countries rather than regions since regions within countries do not usually have the necessary sovereignty. Nevertheless, the analysis may shed some light on the politics of intra-national migrant employment. We should, of course, recall that migrant employment will tend to be socially efficient from a global perspective. However, from the parochial perspective of the 'optimal tariff' there is a case to be considered. In what follows we switch to an algebraic presentation.

Since the respective capital stocks are assumed to be fixed we may write the production functions for S and H respectively as:[11]

$$Y_S = A(L_S - X)^a \qquad 0 \leqslant a \leqslant 1 \qquad (10.1)$$

$$Y_H = B(L_H + X)^b \qquad 0 \leqslant b \leqslant 1 \qquad (10.2)$$

where Y denotes GDP, L denotes the native labour force and X the volume of migrant employment in H. The per capita income of the remaining population in S may be written as

$$GNP_S^* = \frac{Y_S + cXW_H (1 - T_H)}{L_S - X + Z_S} \qquad (10.3)$$

where W_H is the wage rate in H. T_H is the tax rate and c < 1 is the remittance factor. Z reflects the possibility that profits might not necessarily accrue to labour. The per capita income of the native population in H may be written as

$$GNP^*_H = \frac{Y_H - XW_H (1-T_H)}{L_H + Z_H} \qquad (10.4)$$

However, in what follows our concern is with $\triangle GNP^*_S$ of the change in the aggregate net per capita income status of those remaining in the source region which may be written as:[12]

$$\triangle GNP^*_S = A\frac{[(L_S-X)^a - L_S^a + Xa(1-T_s)^{a-1}] + cX(1-T_H)bB(L_H+X)^{b-1}}{L_S - X + Z_S} \qquad (10.5)$$

Equation (10.5) takes account of the fact that wage rates will equal the respective marginal labour products and the diagrammatic analysis of the previous section has been generalised to take account of differential taxation. Thus it is important to take account of the fact that when a migrant worker pays taxes to the host region this is at the expense of the taxes that he would otherwise have paid to the authorities in the source region. This creates an additional source of divergence between the private and social interest since migrant workers (and migrants generally) will look to post-tax wage differentials between H and S when what matters socially is the pre-tax wage.

The problem under consideration is how to maximise $\triangle GNP^*_S$ under the assumption that over the relevant range the post-tax wage in H is sufficiently high to attract migrant workers from S.[13] This may be determined by differentiating equation (10.5) with respect to X, setting the result to zero and solving for X^*. Unfortunately, the resulting expression is highly non-linear in X and X^* does not have an analytical solution. However, a number of fairly obvious properties of X^* may be identified. Clearly, the higher is c, the greater will be the benefits at the margin of migrant workers' remittances. Likewise, the greater is B (i.e., the richer the host country) and the lower the tax rate (T_H) the greater will be the marginal remittance, ceteris paribus. In all of these cases, it will be in the interests of S to foster a larger volume of migrant workers, in which case X^* will vary directly with c and B and inversely with T_H. If tax rates in S are higher this will mean that a greater proportion of earnings accrue to the state and so to the remaining population at large. Therefore, the social income foregone in S through migrant employment will vary directly with the tax rate in which case X^* will also vary inversely with T_S.

To consider the implications of different production functions for X^* equation (10.5) is solved numerically where the basic assumptions are

$A = 100$, $B = 154$, $L_S = 100$, $L_H = 100$, $a = 0.6$, $b = 0.7$,
$T_S = 0.3$, $T_H = 0.3$, $c = 0.25$, $Z = 0$.

These assumptions imply that when $X = 0$ the post-tax wage rate in H is

175

twice that in S. Under these assumptions equation (10.5) is at a maximum when X = 33, implying that optimality is achieved when a third of the work force of S operates as migrant workers in H.[14] When a was raised to 0.62 from 0.6[15] X^* fell from 33 to 24. In this case, there are two separate effects to consider. First the marginal product of labour in S will be higher when X = 0 [16] so that the tax revenues foregone by S through migrant employment will be greater. Secondly, however, the surplus foregone will tend to decline at a slower rate with X.[17] The former effect would tend to reduce X^* while the opposite would tend to happen through the second effect. In the above example, the former effect happens to dominate the second effect.

The converse result holds when b is raised from 0.7 to 0.72[18] and X^* rises from 33 to 42. In this case, there are two reinforcing effects. First, the greater is b the greater will be wage rates in H and the greater will be remittances at the margin. Secondly, the rate of decline of wage rates in H with respect to X will be slower. Both of these factors would suggest that X^* varies directly with b.

Sharing the surplus

The assumption so far has been that migrant workers now operating in H did not consume any of the surplus (i.e., profits on capital or tax revenues) while they were operating in S. This implies that workers and capitalists are dichotomised in the case of consumption out of profits. An alternative assumption might be that workers have equal shares in the capital stock and consume equal shares of the surplus. It may easily be shown that in this case the remaining population in S is better off in the presence of migrant employment assuming that the migrant workers do not take their capital with them or transfer the profits from S to H, assumptions which are likely to apply in the case of temporary migration.

Figure 10.2 largely repeats the left-hand side of Figure 10.1. Since et = ta it follows that etnd = ead. The previous wage share of the migrant workers (rc) was rydc and their profit share would have been ymnd. It follows, therefore, that when rc of the labour force become migrant workers the loss of surplus ysd is less than the previous consumption of these workers since ymnd > ysd. In other words, under the assumptions made the remaining population is better off (even before the remittances are considered) since it partakes of the rewards to capital that previously accrued to the migrant workers. Under such circumstances, the remaining population in S would have no reason to object to migrant employment (and migration in general); on the contrary.[19]

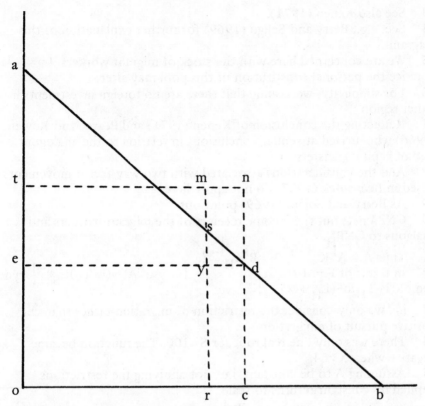

Figure 10.2 The source country

Concluding remarks

The previous discussion emphasises the sensitivity of the analysis to the assumptions about factor ownership. There are of course many further avenues that warrant exploration such as dynamic considerations, terms of trade effects, etc. Pearce and Rowan (1966), Jones (1967) explored some of the welfare implications of integrating capital and trade movements. A yet more general model would add labour movements to this list for which the discussion in this chapter might serve as a starting point.

Notes

1   See e.g., Paine (1974) and Abadan-Unat et.al., (1976).
2   This problem is ambiguous in certain respects to the 'optimal tariff' on capital movements. See e.g., Kemp (1962) and Beenstock (1977).

177

3   See also Kenen (1971).

4   See, e.g., Berry and Seligo (1969) for further explanation of this diagram.

5   We are concerned here with the stock of migrant workers. In practice the personal constitution of this pool may alter.

6   For simplicity, we assume that there are no foreign investments in either region.

7   Reflecting the conclusion of Kenen (1971) and Pearce and Rowan (1966) who arrived at similar conclusions in relation to the analogous case of capital transfers.

8   And the considerations associated with two way factor movements raised in Beenstock (1977) do not apply here.

9   As Berry and Soligo (1969) point out.

10   GNP_S^* nets out the income receipts of the migrant workers and is analogous to GNP_H^*.

11   Thus $A = A^l K_S^{1-a}$, $B = B^l K_H^{1-b}$.

12   In terms of Fig. 10.1, $A[\qquad\qquad] = ysd$, $ADa(1-T_S)L_S^{a-l} = ryde$ and $cX(1-T_H)bS(L_H + X)^{b-l} = wxvu$.

13   i.e. we only consider the restriction of migration rather than the positive pursuit of emigration.

14   There was only one real root for $S \leqslant 100$. The function became negative when $X > 64$.

15   Assuming A to be constant, i.e., not applying the restrictions implied by constant returns to scale.

16   Since $\dfrac{d}{da}(AaL_S^{a-l}) = AL_S^{a-l}(1+a) > 0$.

17   Since on Fig. 10.1 the angle yds will be smaller.

18   Holding H constant.

19   Assuming equal capital ownership, no remittances and where emigrants take their capital with them, the welfare of the remaining population would not be affected assuming constant returns to scale. The per capita income of the eventual remaining population before emigration is

$$-\frac{(L_S - X)}{L_S} A^l K_S^{1-a} L_S^a$$

while after emigration it is

$$A^l \left(\frac{(L_S - X) K_S}{L_S}\right)^{1-a} (L_S - X)^a = \frac{L_S - X}{L_S} A^l K_S^{1-a} L_S^a$$

If there are increasing returns to scale, emigration leaves the remaining population worse off.

Bibliography

Abadan-Unat, N. et al., (1976), *Turkish Workers in Europe, 1960-1975;*
E. J. Brill, Leiden.

Beenstock, M. (1977), Policies Towards International Direct Investment:
a Neoclassical Reappraisal, *Economic Journal* 86, September.

Berry, R. A. and R. Soligo, (1969), Some Welfare Aspects of
International Migration, *Journal of Political Economy* 77, September/
October.

Jones, R. W. (1967), International Capital Movements and the Theory
of Tariffs and Trade, *Quarterly Journal of Economics* 81, February.

Kemp, M. C. (1962), The Benefits and Costs of Private Investment from
Abroad: Comment, *Economic Record* 38.

Kenen, P. B. (1971), Migration, the Terms of Trade and Economic
Welfare in the Source Country, Chapter 11 in J. N. Bhagwati et al.,
(eds), *Trade, Balance of Payments and Growth;* North Holland
Publishing Company, Amsterdam.

Paine, S. (1974), *Exporting Workers: the Turkish Case,* Cambridge
University Press.

Pearce, I. F. and Rowan, D. C. (1966), A Framework for Research into
the Real Effects of International Capital Movements, in T. Bogiotti
(ed), *Essays in Honour of Macro Fanno;* Cedam, Padova.

Index

Abadan-Unat, N., et al, 177, 179
Ahluwalia, M. S., 103
Aid/external assistance, 69, 71,
    72-74, chap. 4 passim
Alang-alang, 155
Anaemia, 9, 15, 16, 94
    and productivity, 26-29, 32
Animateur/seconuriste, 52
Arndt, H. W., 105
Ascariasis, 29

Bali, 94, 110, 111, 115
Bamako, 51, 65, 80, 91
Bangladesh, 144
Basic needs, 2, 5-6, 8, chap. 3
    in Mali, chap. 4
Basta, S., vi
Basta, S., and Churchill, A., 27,
    28, 33, 104
Becker, G., 16, 33
Beenstock, M., 153, 178, 179
Belavady, B., 26, 33
Bengkulu, 154
Berg, A., vi, 22, 33
Beriberi, 22
Berry, A., and R. Soligo, 179,
    178, 179
Boserup, E., 161
Brain drain, 170
Brozek, J. et al, 33

Calories, 6, 7, 15, 16, 17, 18,
    22, chap. 5
    and productivity, 23-26, 32
Cassava, chap. 5
Central Bank of Mali, 49, 50
Chad, 91

Chambers, R., 135, 142
Chenery, H., 12
Collier, P., 162, 168
Collier, W. L., et al, 141, 142
Co-operatives
    in Mali, 51
Correa, H., 33
Corruption, 149, 152
Cretinism, 22

Dapice, D., vi, 103
Davies, G., 136
Doctors, 7
Donges, J. B., et al, 141, 153
Dozier, C. L., 135, 136, 137, 142,
    149, 153
Drugs, 9
    in Mali, 47, 49, 51, 61, 63, 69,
    78
    tax policy, 88-89
Dysentery, 31

Edmunson, 18, 33, 94, 101, 104
Education, 122
    and basic needs, chap. 3
Employment, 4, 22, 120-121
    urban, 4
    elasticity, 112, 113
    agricultural, 112, 113
Esmara, H., 111
Exchange rate, 119, 121, 123, 152

Far Eastern Economic Review, 10
Farmer, B. H., 135, 136, 142
Fields, G. S., 162, 168
F.A.O., 96
FELDA, 136

Fitzgerald, D. P., 136, 142, 149, 153
France, 69

Gao, 91
Gardener, G. W., 28, 33
Goiter, 22
Golladay, Fred, vi
Green Revolution, 112, 151
Guest-workers, 12

Haemoglobin, 18, 27, 28, 29, 32
Haemotocrit, 18, 29
Harberger, A., 15, 33, 35
Harris, J. and M. Todaro, 11, 12, chap. 9
Health
  planning, 2, chap. 3, 53-59
  statistics, 3
  as investment, 9
  curative, 9, 63-64, 72, 77, 79 86-87
  preventive, 9, 56, 63-64, 66, 72, 77, 79, 86-87
  in Mali, chap. 4
Hong Kong, 122, 151
Hookworm, 18, 29
Horakova, E., 135, 136, 142, 149, 153

Income distribution, 4-5, 35, 173
  in Mali, 90-92
  in Indonesia, 118, 139
INCORA (Columbia), 140
Indonesia, 10, 11, chaps. 6-7
Involution (agricultural), 112, 122
Iodine deficiency, 22, 95
Iron (see anaemia), 17, 18, 19, 22, 27, 28, chap. 5
Irwin, M. I., et al, 33

Jakarta, 122
Japan, 122, 151
Java, 10, 94, 96, 110-111-115, 124

143-145, 151, 154
Johnson, W. S., 153
Jones, G., 141
Jones, R., 177, 179

Kalimantan, 9, 111, 146, 148
Karyadi, D. and S. Basta, 26, 104
Kayes, 52, 90
Keita, 51, 53
Kelantan State Land Development Authority (KSLDA), 136
Kemp, M. C., 177, 179
Kenen, P. B., 178, 179
Keys, et al, 23, 24, 33
Kirschmann, J. D., 104
Korea, 122, 151
Kraut, H. A. and Muller, E. A., 33

Lampung, 154
Land settlement, 124-141, chap. 7
Latham and Brooks, 24, 25, 26, 33
Lewis, W. A., 4, 12
Life expectancy, 6, 7, 22
  and basic needs, chap. 3
Literacy, 7, 8, 30, 31, 122
  and basic needs, chap. 3

Maarten, D. C., et al, 33
MacAndrews, C., 142
Madura, 94, 96, 110, 115
Malaria, 31, 125, 146
Malaysia, 144
Malenbaum, W., 30, 31, 33
Malawi, 59
Mali, 1, 9, chap. 4
Malnutrition, 94-95
Maternities, 9, 52, 78
Mazumdar, D., 12
McGarry, M., vi
Metabolism, 17-18, 20
Migration, 1, 2, 11, 113-115
  rural-urban, 11, chap. 9
  international, 12, chap. 10
Mopti, 48, 52, 65, 90, 91

Morawetz, D., 12
Morbidity, 20, 21, 38
Myrdal, G., 135

Nain, D., 104
Nelson, M., 134, 137, 142, 148,
    149, 153
Niacin, 17, chap. 5
Nutrition, 6, 8, 9, chap. 2, 5
    and basic needs, chap. 3
Nye, P. H. and D. J. Greenland,
    161

Paine, S., 177, 180
Pearce, I. and D. Rowan, 177,
    178, 179
Pelzer, K. J., 142, 161
Penny, D. H. and Gittinger, J. P.,
    142
Pertamina, 119
Pharmacie d'Approvisionnement,
    63, 79
Pharmacie Populaire, 49, 50, 51,
    78
Philippines, 28, 149
Phillips, Tony, vi
Pioneering, 125, 128-129, 130,
    135, 137
Popkin, B. et al, 28, 29, 33
Popkin, B. and Lim-Ybanes, M.,
    28, 33
Population, 110
    in Indonesia, 110-111, 113-
        115, 124, 126, 145, 146
    per doctor etc, 7, 41-44
Poverty, 5, 6, 118, 124
    absolute, 2, 3, 8, 144
    measurement, 9, 93
    line, 10, 94, 103, 118
Productivity
    and health, 8, chap. 2, 36, 39
    and nutrition, 16, 72
Protein, 16, 17, 22, 41-44, chap. 5

Rawls, J., 5, 12
Recurrent costs, 9, 48, 72-74
Redistribution with growth, 4-5, 35
Riboflavin, 17, chap. 5
Rice, 5, chap. 5, 118
Rose, C. S. and Gyorgy, P   104
Rural sector, 4, 11, chap. 9
Ruthenberg, H., 161

Sabot, R. H., 12
Sanitation, 6, 15, 77
    and basic needs, chap. 3
Satyanarayana, K. et al, 33
Schistosomiasis, 18, 29, 30
Segou, 91
Self-help, 9, 51, 79
Selowsky and Reutlinger, 15, 33
Shifting cultivation, 11, chap. 8
Sikasso, 49, 51, 52, 79, 80, 91
Spencer, J. E., 161
Spurr, G. B., et al, 29, 33
Srikantia, S. G., 21, 33
Stongyloidiasis, 29, 30
Streeten, P., vi, 12
Strout, A., 151
Sulawesi, 111, 146
Sumatra, 1, 94, 111, 112, 113, 114,
    154
Sukarno, 131, 151
Synergy, 18, 40, 43

Taiwan, 122, 151
Tandon, B. N., et al, 34
Thiamin, 17, chap. 5
Todaro, M., chap. 9
    see Harris
Transmigration, 10, chaps. 6-7
Trichuriasis, 29, 30
Turnham, D. and I. Jaeger, 12
Two-gap Theory, 3-4

Vitamin
    B1, 22
    A, 22, chap. 5

C, chap. 5
B12, 95
D, 95
E, 95

Wafa, S. H., 136, 142
Wall Street Journal, 10
Water supply, 7, 8, 9, 15, 77
    and basic needs, chap. 3
Weisbrod, B. A. and T. W.
    Helminiak, 29, 30, 34
Wells, 51, 69, 78
White, B., 141, 153
World Bank, vi, 5, 8, 12
World Health Organisation,
    18, 34, 94